Black Seed Oil

The Comprehensive Guide on Benefit of Black Seed Oil

(The Proven Healing Health Benefits Used as a Natural Supplement)

Raymond Murphy

Published By **Bengion Cosalas**

Raymond Murphy

Black Seed Oil: The Comprehensive Guide on Benefit of Black Seed Oil (The Proven Healing Health Benefits Used as a Natural Supplement)

ISBN 978-1-7775767-5-2

No part of this guidebook shall be reproduced in any form without permission in writing from the publisher except in the case of brief quotations embodied in critical articles or reviews.

Legal & Disclaimer

The information contained in this book is not designed to replace or take the place of any form of medicine or professional medical advice. The information in this book has been provided for educational & entertainment purposes only.

The information contained in this book has been compiled from sources deemed reliable, and it is accurate to the best of the Author's knowledge; however, the Author cannot guarantee its accuracy and validity and cannot be held liable for any errors or omissions. Changes are periodically made to this book. You must consult your doctor or get professional medical advice before using any of the suggested remedies, techniques, or information in this book.

Table Of Contents

Chapter 1: Black Seed Oil

Today we are seeing people embracing the natural methods of Treating various diseases, ailments and concerns because the allopathic/conventional medicines mostly come up with side effects Allopathic refers to the method by where medical doctors as well as other health care specialists (such as pharmacists, nurses as well as therapy professionals) deal with symptoms and ailments with radiation, medications, or surgical procedures. In the end, all, patients will be not aware of the side effects they suffer.

This book will take you more than you could ever imagine or anticipate what black seed can do. In this book you will also learn how to use Black seed in various forms (Oil, powder, raw seeds) to solve several health challenges/illnesses.

Certainly, a lot of people who used black seeds previously with no or no results use it in a wrong way because many vendors/sellers do not sell black seed with prescription/instruction on how to use. This guide will provide an extremely helpful reference that will help you to be confident of the proper way to utilize this amazing product.

The seeds of black cumin were used for treating different ailments throughout the centuries throughout the world, particularly within the Mediterranean, Middle East, as well as India. The Europeans and many other countries have also utilized the black cumin seeds to make natural remedies.

It is evident that it is evident that black cumin seeds are powerful and are capable of treating any disease other than death. It is possible to treat any kind of chronic ailments by following the suggestions mentioned earlier.

Most people say they've tried the black cumin seed, or oil in the treatment of illnesses, yet the issue remained exactly the same. It does not suggest that black cumin seeds does not work in curing these ailments. There is simply a ignorance about how to utilize the seeds of black cumin. Keep in mind that if you do make a mistake in using it your results might not be satisfying.

The following tips will enable you to understand the most effective application of black cumin seeds and the oil of black cumin seed.

1. Make sure you use it in accordance with the instructions. Different diseases call for diverse forms of the black seed. As an example, there are People use black cumin seeds as a remedy for illnesses, and require the oil of black cumin. Be aware that the black cumin oil as well as black cumin seeds are derived from the same plant i.e. Nigella Sativa, but they have distinct features. This is why it is essential to apply the oil extracted from black seeds for this disease. It requires certain characteristics in the black seed oil, and reverse.

You can also use other compounds:

A common occurrence among those who are prone to only considering Nigella Sativa as the remedy, however they do not combine it with other substances needed to ease the pain of some diseases. Keep in mind that sometimes, black cumin seeds don't perform well on its own, but mixing it with beneficial compounds like honey, warm water as well as sesame oil and olive oil cinnamon, fenugreek. could be beneficial. This is why you must make use of all natural herbal remedies or compounds that are as a mixture or paste, to get an immediate cure for ailments.

Usage Duration:

A few people are saying that the treatment is not effective. It won't help in the event that you don't take it for a long enough time. Everybody knows that overcoming the smallest of ailments is usually a process that takes two to three months, sometimes longer. But, most people only take this for a few days or weeks, and then think that it's not effective. The key is to recognize that it is a process that takes time to treat a illness. Additionally, researchers have stated in their papers on research studies Nigella sativa that it could require between two and three months for an illness to be eliminated making use of the black cumin seed. Furthermore, it is likely to yield the most effective results in the case of a long time period, which is six months in various diseases.

Black Seed Products:

Because black seeds are considered to be the as the best treatment for any diseases, a lot of researchers are studying it in order to discover more about its therapeutic benefits. To date, many illnesses have been successfully treated by using black seeds as well as oil. They believe that there's more. Because it's becoming an effective treatment for various diseases and ailments, doctors are carrying out tests to create different kinds of products with Black seeds.

An IMPORTANT NOTE A QUICK NOTE: I believe it's vital to provide the reader with information on the beginning in this book regarding Black seeds oil during pregnancy.

Do you think that Black Seed oil can be employed during pregnancy?

The pregnancy is among the most serious concerns that must be taken care of until baby is born. There is a lot of pregnant women consume black seeds when they are pregnant and cite to the phrase, "It cures all diseases except death." But the women who are pregnant should recognize that pregnancy isn't an illness that can be treated with the oil of black seeds or other grains. The most highly recommended method is to use black cumin seeds during pregnancy. If you do, there will most likely result in the abortion. Additionally, the following issues can arise:

*A premature child delivery

*Contraction of the uterus following the birth

*The odds of children surviving decrease

If the child does survive, it could be suffering from ailment.

*chronic illnesses

Urinary and uterus diseases can occur following pregnancy.

So, pregnant women must be advised not to consume the black cumin seeds as it can be harmful for the baby and mother.

After the birth the mother may begin drinking black seed oil in order for increased the production of milk. Also, after baby's birth, taking a few drops of oil from the black cumin seeds to the newborn will assist the baby grow healthier. It is the ideal way to use Nigella Sativa to help with the development of your baby.

WHAT IS BLACK SEED OIL

If ancient Egyptian monarchs, European queens, religious prophets, and contemporary scientists meet on a topic and discuss it, it's worth checking out. Even though we've got more access to information than previously, there is many lessons to be learned from our past.

Beginning with Hippocrates and Cleopatra, through the reign of King Tut and the other civilizations that followed, the only thing they all had in common was their belief on a specific plant. The herb in question is nothing more than the black seeds.

We decided to learn about it ourselves and reveal the many benefits that are lauded by the oil of black seeds.

Black seeds can be identified by a myriad of names, based on the region that you are. Below are a handful of the most popular ones the plant is known by:

Chapter 2: The Seeds & The Powder Black Cumin Seeds

In addition to Nigella Sativa oil, the seeds of Nigella Sativa (also called black cumin) comprise a variety of useful sources. It's a source of unsaturated fats. Here are the two main unsaturated fatty acids that are found in the seeds of Nigella Sativa 58 percent Linoleic acid, which is Omega-6 , 23 percent Oleic acid.

These saturated fats found include 14 The percentage of saturated fatty acids is 14 Palmitic acid and 3 percent Stearic acid, black cumin seed, the powder and oil, contain 15 amino acids, which comprise the nine most essential amino acids that are essential to a healthy eating habits. The structure of Nigella isativa reveals the precise understanding of this miraculous plant. Due to these nutrients the seed has been utilized in the treatment of ailments.

different ailments. Researchers have demonstrated that black cumin seeds can help with anti-cancer effects and also anti-acids.

As a summary, Black Seeds contains over 44 Super minerals. These are Aliphatic

Aspartic Acid

Copper

Esters

Glycosides

Limonene

Melatonin

Mucilage

Phytoestrogens Resins

Steroids

Terpene

Alkaloids

Beta Sitosterol

Carvone

Eicosanoid acid

Fatty Acids

Iron

Linoleic Acid

Monosaccharide

Myristic Acid

Saponins

Stigmasterol

Terpenoids

Zinc

Amino Acids

Calcium

Citronellol

Quinine

Essential Oil

Fixed Oil

Leucine

Lysine or

Monoterpene

Protein

Stearic Acid

Tannins

Thymoquinone

The vitamins and minerals in the black seed oil allow it to be an all-purpose natural cure to treat just about all things. The black seed oil can be used for:

* Anodyne is a painkiller that heals

* Anthelmintic This is the process of removing Parasite worms as well as other internal parasites out of the body and does not cause any harm to the person or host (without any adverse side consequences)

Anti-arthritic relieves the signs of Arthritis It also cures Arthritis It also helps prevent Arthritis

* Anti-asthmatic. Relieves all signs of Asthma and offers cures.

* Anti-bacterial - Destroys bacteria completely

* Antibiotic All-body - kills or destroys microorganisms

Anti-cancer works against Cancer It also stops and wards off cancer

* Anticoagulant, which has effects of slowing down or preventing the coagulation process of blood

* Anti-dandruff clears and stops the growth of dandruff

* Anti-diabetic - - Treats Diabetics It also prevents and treats every symptom.

* Anti-diarrheal - Treats Diarrhea

* Anti-fungal, which stops from the development of yeasts as well as other fungal organisms.

Anti-hematoma can help treat a swelling that is solid and blood that has clotted within tissues.

* Anti-histamines treat allergies.

* Anti-hypertensive. Balances and lowers blood pressure

* Anti-inflammatory - decreases the inflammation (redness or swelling) and the sensation of pain) throughout the body.

* Anti-lithic prevents the growth of or development of calculi as of the urinary tract.

* Anti-malarial - Treats malaria effectively

* Antimicrobial, eliminates microorganisms, including viruses, bacteria and the fungi

* Anti-nociceptive is the act or method of preventing the perception of sensitive or painful stimuli by sensory neurons.

* Anti-oxidants are compounds that stop or reduce the damage caused to cells through free radicals. They are unstable substances that your body creates due to stressors and environmental pressures. Antioxidants are substances that combat free radicals that are present in the body. Free radicals are substances which could cause harm when their concentrations become elevated within the body. They're connected to a myriad of diseases like heart disease, diabetes as well as cancer.

* Anti-parasitic effective for treating parasites

* Anti-protozoal to treat diseases caused by protozoa

* Anti-pyretic - Relieves/cures the symptoms of fever.

* Anti-septic, which stops the spread of microorganisms that cause disease.

Anti-spasmodic is a medication that reduces, stops, or reduces the frequency of spasms in muscles, particularly the ones caused by smooth muscle, such as those found in the intestinal wall.

* Anti-tumor: stopping or inhibiting the development and growth of cancerous tumors anticancer drugs"antitumor activities.

* Anti-viral - treatment effective against viruses.

* Appetizer - is served to serve as an appetizer

* Aromatic-black seeds have aromas and can either be pleasant or unpleasing (depends on the individual)

* Brain Enhancer - Continuous use of black seeds improves memory and the brain.

* Carminative - relieves flatulence.

* Cytotoxic is a treatment for cancer. It can also be used to treat different disorders, including Rheumatoid arthritis as well as multiple sclerosis.

* Deoxidant is the process of removing the harmful chemical (such as toxin or poison) or the influence of it from your body. Renders (a harmful substance) harmless.

* Digestive is a supplement that assists in the digestion process of food.

* Emmenagogue helps to stimulate or increase the flow of menstrual blood

* Expectorant is a medicine that patients are able to take when they suffer from an asthmatic cough which produces mucus.

* Febrifuge, a drug that is used to lower the severity of fever.

* Galactagogue helps boost the the production of milk from breasts.

* Hepatoprotective, which prevents the damage to the liver.

* Anti-Hypertensive, which treats hypertension effectively.

* Hypoglycemic-related - Treats Low blood sugar

* Immunity Booster Immunity system is a complex set made up of proteins and cells which guards against infections. When your immune system is not functioning properly and weak, it's easy to become sick. The Black Seeds do an excellent job and boost the immune system to help not to fall sick easily.

* Insecticidal-Capable to kill insects and control the growth of insects

* Laxative that helps ease constipation

* Lithotripsic helps in breaking down or eliminating stones in the kidneys or bladder

* Memory Enhancer - can help improve memory

* Ophthalmic is helpful in treating various eye disorders

* Purgative is an effective laxative when it is used according to the proper manner.

* Stimulant that assists the body to improve its performance and become smart

* Stomachic - encouraging the appetite or helping with digestion

* Therapeutic helps with the healing process of many diseases

* Thermogenics - increase metabolism, boost the burning of fat and decrease the appetite.

* Tonic provides the feeling of vitality or a sense of well-being

* Vermifuge: kills and eliminates parasite worms from your body.

BLACK SEED CAN EFFECTIVELY TREAT THE BELOW HEALTH CONDITIONS:

* Ascaris

* Abscess

* Acid Reflux

* Acne

* Allergy

* Alzheimer

* Anemia

* Anxiety

* Arthritis

* Asthma

* Autoimmune Diseases

* Bee Stings

* Bloating

* Blocked Nose

* Brain Cancer

* Breast Cancer

* Bronchitis

* Burns

* Candidiasis

* Carbuncle

* Cervical Cancer

* Chest Congestion

* Colic

* Colon Cancer

* Constipation

* Cough

* Dandruff

* Debility

* Dementia

* Depression

* Diabetes

* Diarrhea

* Digestive Disorder

* Dizziness

* Dry Lips

* Earache

* Eczema

* Epilepsy

* Eye Diseases

* Fatigue

* Fever

* Flatulence

* Flu

* Fungal Nails

* Gallstones

* Gum Diseases

* Headache

* Heart Attack

* Hepatitis

* High Blood P Pressure

* HIV AIDS

* Indigestion

Chapter 3: How To Use For Different Health Challenges

This article will teach you the best ways to utilize Black Seeds, Black Seed Oil as well as the Black Seed Powder in order to treat different health issues. Additionally, we have included additional compounds and oils to mix with the black seeds for a more efficient results. Carefully read and note the instructions/procedures. Other compound ingredients that are suitable for use in conjunction with Black seed include Aniseed, apple Cider Vinegar Azadiracnta Indica, Basil Cinnamon, Coconut Oil, Cumin Garlic, Garlic and Golden Bamboo Honey Mint, Milk, Nutmeg, Olive, Saffron and Squilla Maritima. Yogurt, Sugarcane, Wheat and more.

HEALTH CONDITION: HYPERTENSION

What to Use: Garlic Cloves, Black seeds (Raw)/powder Oil of Black Seeds Oil and Garlic Cloves

The best way to use high blood pressure i.e. hypertension is among the reasons that patients suffer from diseases such as heart attacks, strokes and kidney problems. There are a variety of causes that can lead to high blood pressure. The most common causes of hypertension include:

*Excessive stress

There is less blood supply as a result of shrinking blood vessels

High intake of salt

Excessive consumption of alcohol

*Repeated use of caffeine

Hereditary and hormonal reasons

The utilization of black cumin seeds can be beneficial in resolving hypertension concerns. Based on recent research conducted about Nigella Sativa it is believed that there are 15 amino acids and alkaloids carbohydrate, as well as dietary fiber, within the black cumin seeds. Research also suggests that the amino acid composition can help regulate the blood flow in veins.

But, to do that, it is essential to know the ways that black cumin seeds could help to treat hypertension effectively. Below are some suggestions for making use of black cumin seeds that are worth considering to address the issues you are facing:

The black cumin grains daily will help to maintain the flow of blood throughout the our body. It is recommended to use the oil from Nigella Sativa also. In order to treat hypertension, consume a teaspoon of oil from black cumin with an alcoholic beverage at breakfast. This will work better by including two garlic cloves to the previously mentioned method. Smash the cloves, and then take out the liquid. Mix in 1 teaspoon of Black seeds oil. Drink this mixture in the morning and at night.

Nigella Sativa oil can additionally used to relax your body as well as helping to keep the nerves relaxed. To manage hypertension, it's crucial that you provide adequate relaxation the body.

In order to do that, apply the Black Cumin Seed Oil to the body, and then expose it to sunlight for around 30 minutes. Repeating the exercise at least each week then you'll become free of the high blood pressure issues. If you start following these basic techniques, you'll see the benefits.

You will notice a positive change inside the outside of you, which means after the time of a couple of months, you'll become free of hypertension issues.

The minimum recommended duration is each day for 3 months for full cure.

HEALTH CONDITION: FOR HEPATITIS D

How to use What to Use: Oil from Black Seeds

What to do: Include Black Cumin Oil in daily eating habits.

Minimal Duration: Recommended to use each day for 3 months

HEALTH CONDITION: DIABETES

What to Use: Raw Black Seeds

The best way to use it: drink 20 milliliters of decoction from Black Cumin seed. Drink it every day. Do it for a full month, and then see how it works.

How do I create Black Seed Decoction? The raw black seeds are boiled in water. It is possible to add 50cl of water or 30g of black seeds. Boil for some minutes. Sift the liquid. Drink it when it's cool, or warm.

Minimum Time Limit: Try for a month before going for a follow-up. Keep using if you notice an improvement or change until the happy with your results.

HEALTH CONDITION: PARALYSIS.

How is the best way to use: Oil from black seeds, milk

How to Use: Put 3 ml of black cumin seed oil to 30 ml of milk. Drink it 3 times per day.

The minimum recommended duration is 1 Month

HEALTH CONDITION: ARTHRITIS

How to use What to Use: Vinegar, Black Seed oil Honey, Black seed oil

What to Mix Make a Mixture of Vinegar with Black Seed oil, and honey in a 2:1:4 ratio. Use 2 tablespoons every daily.

For example, 5ml Vinegar plus 3ml or 2.5ml Black seed oil and 10ml of honey. Use 2 teaspoonfuls of the mixture two times a day. Both at night and in the morning.

Minimum Recommended Duration: 8 weeks

HEALTH CONDITION: STOMACH PROBLEMS

How to use What to Use: Black Seed Oil and ginger juice

How to use: Create the mixture consisting of Black Cumin seed oil and Ginger juice, in a ratio of 2:1. Consume 2 tablespoons every day. E.G 5ml of black seeds oil mixture with 2.5ml the juice of ginger.

Minimum Duration Recommended: Use until symptoms disappears

HEALTH CONDITION: EYE DISEASES

What to Use: Black Seed Oil, Carrot Juice.

How to use: Prepare the mixture by mixing 1/2 1 teaspoon Black Cumin seed oil in cup of juice from carrots. Take it every day twice. Take note that the juice you make use of should be a 100% pure carrot juice. It is recommended to grind the carrot yourself and then get the juice.

Minimum Time-Recommended: Use up to 2 months for a full treatment.

LEUCORRHOEA

HEALTH CONDITION: LEUCORRHOEA

Which Form is best for you to use What Form is best to use? Raw Black Seed or Mint Leaves

What to do: Use 1 teaspoon of seeds from Black Cumin as well as a couple of Mint leaves. Cook them in 1 glass of water. Take it once per each day.

The recommended minimum duration is between 2 and 3 months

HEALTH CONDITION: FOR SCANTY MENSES

Optional: Add Black Cumin Seed oil to Honey.

Which form is the best one to use the best form is black seed powder organic honey, milk

What to use: Mix two teaspoons Black Cumin seed powder oil together with the exact amount of Honey. Drink it along with warm Milk two times the course of a single morning.

The recommended minimum duration is between 1 and 2 weeks.

Chapter 4: Health Condition For Cancer

Which Form is best for use the best is: Black Seed Oil, grape juice

What to use: Black seeds with thymoquinone and anti-oxidant qualities provide powerful scavenger capabilities. They're not just useful to treat a myriad of illnesses, but are an important ingredient in slowing of tumor cell growth. Their capability to stop the growth of cancer is so remarkable that numerous doctors have declared that it is a viable natural treatment option for cancer.

Drink a cup Grape juice. Include 3ml of Black Cumin seed oil to it. Take it 2 times per every day.

Minimum Duration: You should do this for a period of weeks, while you seek a doctor's note to observe an improvement.

HEALTH CONDITION: FOR FATIGUE

What to Use: Seeds, pure orange juice

How to use: Make the decoction from Black Cumin seeds. Include 5 ml to a cup of Orange juice. Take a glass of juice every daily. (Boil the seeds in water. Combine 5ml of it's liquid into a glass of juice from an orange)

Minimum duration recommended use as necessary.

HEALTH CONDITION: KIDNEY DISEASES

The seeds of black cumin are crushed into a powder. Add 300 g of it in 600 ml Honey. Consume 1 teaspoon at least twice per daily.

How to Use How to Use Seed powder Original Honey

What to do: Grind the seeds of black cumin to create a powder. Add 300 g of it in 600 ml Honey. Use 1 tsp every daily.

Minimum Time Limit: Everyday for between 2 and 3 months.

HEALTH CONDITION: TO BOOST IMMUNE SYSTEM

What to use What to Use: Black Seed Oil, garlic cloves

What to use: Black Cumin Seed Oil is an excellent immune boosting oil. It boosts the ability of your body to combat external elements that cause diseases. It is also possible to use black seeds to enhance your immunity, thus enhancing the body's defense system and ability to fight off the harmful bacteria. Because the majority of modern diseases are caused by

My swelling, black seeds are an ideal herb for treating various ailments people are suffering from in the present.

Include half a teaspoon Black Cumin Seed Oil in two crushed garlic cloves to paste. Mix it thoroughly. Drink it regularly.

Minimum Recommended Duration: between 2 and 3 weeks or longer

HEALTH CONDITION: SWELLING

How to use How to use: Oil extracted from Black Seeds

Method of Use Apply black cumin seed oil on the an affected the area. Don't wash the part with soap for at minimum six hours.

Minimal Duration: Use when needed.

HEALTH CONDITION: FOR TUMOR

What is the best way to use it What to Use: Oil from black seeds

What to do: Take a one half teaspoon of black cumin seeds oil daily. You can also apply it on Tumor.

Minimum duration recommended Utilize as needed.

HEALTH CONDITION: FOR HEADACHE

What is the best way to use it How to use: Black Seed Oil

What to Apply: Put black cumin seed oil to your forehead.

Minimum duration recommended: Use whenever it is necessary.

HEALTH CONDITION: FOR HICCUPS

What To Use How to use: Black seed oil milk cream,

How to Use: Take 1 tsp Milk Cream. Mix two drops Black Cumin seed oil in it. Take it 2 times per every day.

Minimal Duration: Recommended until it is fully healed.

HEALTH CONDITION: FOR BALDNESS

What to Use: Black Seed oil

Method of Use Method: Massage your scalp, and hair with Black Cumin seed oil after shampooing your hair.

Minimum Duration Recommend Minimum Duration: 3 to 6 months

HEALTH CONDITION: FOR BRAIN FEVER

How to Use Raw Black seeds

Method of Use: Warm 1 teaspoon of Black Cumin seeds in a saucepan. Take a deep breath and inhale the smoke.

Minimum Time Required: Repeat whenever required

HEALTH CONDITION: FOR STOMACH ACHE

How to Make: Oil from the black seed or milk

What to do: Drink 1 teaspoon of milk with 2 drops Black Cumin seed oil. Do this twice a each day.

Minimum Recommended Duration: 3-8 days.

HEALTH CONDITION: FOR PILES

What To Use Raw seed that is black,

Method of Use To Roast: Take one Tablespoon Black seeds and mix with the same amount of unroasted Black seeds. Blend well, and then take half a teaspoon daily with water.

Minimum Duration Recommendation: Perform every day and watch the improvement.

HEALTH CONDITION: FOR FEVER

How to use for: Oil from black seeds (Lemon Juice) and Lukewarm water

What to do: Drink 1 cup of water that is lukewarm. Mix in lemon juice and Black Cumin seed oil in the ratio 1:1. Take a drink twice per day.

Minimum Duration Recommended: 3 to 5days

HEALTH CONDITION: FOR ASCARIS

How Do You Use? Black Seed oil, vinegar

What you can do: Create the mixture from Black Cumin seed oil and Vinegar at 1:2 proportions. Use 1 teaspoon every day, two times.

Minimum Recommended Duration: 2-weeks to 2 months

HEALTH CONDITION: FOR Kidney STONE

How to Use How to Use Honey

What to Drink To Drink: Consume half tsp black Cumin oil in one cup of water that is lukewarm. Add 1 tsp honey to the mixture. Drink it twice daily.

Take care not to eat Tomatoes, Spinach and Curry Leaves.

The recommended minimum duration is between 2 and 3 months

HEALTH CONDITION: FOR EPILEPSY

How to use The Original Honey, the Oil from black seeds Also, Lukewarm water

Method of Use Make a mixture of 2 ml honey and 1 ml of black cumin seed oil and 10ml of lukewarm water. Consume it two times a day.

Beware: Avoid eating Guava, Banana and Figs while applying the remedy mentioned above.

Minimum Recommended Duration 3-to-6 months

HEALTH CONDITION: FOR EARS PROBLEMS

How to use What to Use: Raw black seeds, you should also add oil

What to do: Warm 10 grams of Black Cumin seeds in 30ml of water. Then include oil.

Apply it to the ear as a drop when it's bearable hot/lukewarm.

Minimum Time Optimum Utilize as necessary.

BLACK CUMIN

HEALTH CONDITION: FOR DENTAL DISEASES

How to use How to use: Black seed oil

What to Do To Use: Apply oil from Black Cumin on gums or teeth that are painful, or over the tooth.

Minimal Duration use as required.

HEALTH CONDITION: FOR ASTHMA

How to use How to Use It: Black seed oil hot water, coffee

Method of Use: Pour 4 to 5 drops Black Cumin seed oil in boiling water. Take a breath of the steam.

The minimum duration recommended: Use for between 2 and 3 months

OR Use any of the methods below:

Black Cumin Seed Oil (Kalonji Ka Tail in India) can open up the respiratory tract to allow the flow of oxygen through it. It relaxes the tract as well as treats Asthma.

Include 1 tablespoon of Black Cumin Seed Oil in your cup of coffee. Consume it two times over up to 3 days.

OR or 10 drops Black Cumin Seed Oil with up to 4-5 drops of carrier oil. Massage it gently on your chest and the back of your neck over 5-10 minutes.

OR A: Mix one to two teaspoons Black Cumin Seed Oil into hot water. Breathe in the steam for about 10-12 minutes. Repeat this two times per throughout the day.

HEALTH CONDITION: FOR DIARRHEA

How to Use for: Black seed oil Yogurt

Method of Use Make a mixture of half teaspoon Black Cumin seed oil with 50ml of yogurt. Take it every day twice.

Minimum duration recommended Use only when required or needed.

HEALTH CONDITION: FOR BLOCKED NOSE

What is the best way to use it How to use: Black seed oil

Methods to Use: Apply Black Cumin seed oil as Nasal Drop.

Minimal Duration: Use when necessary

HEALTH CONDITION: FOR INSOMNIA

How do I use? Oil from black seeds, milk

How to Use: Put 1 teaspoon Honey and 1/2 1 teaspoon of Black Cumin oil into the milk in a cup that is warm. Take it in the evening and drink it.

Minimal Duration: Use until the result is satisfactory

HEALTH CONDITION: FOR STAMMERING

What to Use:

What to do: Apply the mixture of black seed oil and honey onto the tongue. Make sure to do it at least twice per each day.

Minimum Time Recommend to use until results are acceptable.

HEALTH CONDITION: FOR ABSCESS

How to use: Black seed powder, water

What to do Make a paste of one teaspoon black cumin using a small amount of water. Use it to cover areas of concern for about half an hour.

Minimal Duration: Recommended until you are satisfied with the results

Chapter 5: For Skin Problems

How to use: Black seeds, shampoo Honey, yogurt Sesame oil, vinegar

How to Use: Remedy for Skin Problems

When your face is scratching and breaking out, you should identify the issue before they get worse. There are a variety of causes for skin troubles and can affect your appearance and appearance. Additionally, dry, acne-prone skin, ageing, and skin blister conditions can trigger skin conditions like eczema and psoriasis and even life-threatening conditions.

The effects of these problems can affect your appearance and facial skin. It is therefore vital to think about the necessary steps to prevent issues with your skin at bay. Because black cumin seeds are an all-purpose remedy to treat every ailment, you must apply it to the skin, too. The Nigella sativa plant not only helps with your skin concerns but improves the appearance of your skin. There is no need to purchase other products for your skin and cosmetics in order to enhance your complexion. Black crude oil and cumin seeds can be beneficial in a variety of ways. The following are the primary advantages of using black cumin in skincare the oil from the black seeds shields your skin against wrinkles that are due to the premature ageing process. Additionally, it assists in reducing the appearance of

wrinkles that appear under the wrinkles under the eyes. This is a great solution for dry and flaky skin. Softens and refreshes faster when compared with other creams and cosmetics.

Skin irritation is also eliminated with the help of the black cumin seeds. It also heals the ugly scars created by scratching or rashes on the skin. One of the best things about Nigella Sativa is that it does not just treat dry skin. It also works to treat oily skin. The substances and compounds that are found in Nigella sativa help to keep your skin at a point that oily and dry skin conditions do not become painful. For severe skin problems like eczema and psoriasis and other skin conditions that can severely damage the skin, black seed oil can be considered as a fantastic remedy for relieving the skin of these issues and helps soothe the skin.

Here are a few suggestions on how to make use of black seed oil for diverse skin concerns:

If you're experiencing issues on your scalp, you can solve the problem by adding a few drops of the oil of black seeds in your shampoo. After shower, apply this combination of shampoo and oil in about 10-15 minutes. A daily shower using the same technique will help solve any issues with the skin of your head. Additionally, a mix of yogurt, honey, black seed oil, as well as sesame oil will also help relieve your stress from hair skin.

If you're suffering from face skin issues or you want to brighten your complexion and radiant, you can prepare a paste from honey and black seed. Put it on your skin and let it sit in the sun for around 10-15 minutes throughout the daylight. After that, wash your face. It will give you a silky and shiny feeling on your face.

To maintain your beautiful skin to keep your skin looking beautiful, use dark seeded black powder mixed using olive oil. Apply it to the neck and cover, while exposing it to the sun's rays. But, it is recommended to protect your face by covering it by a slender sheet of cloth. The sun's rays will expose your skin for around 20 minutes. After that, wash off the sun's rays. This won't just solve your acne on the face and itching problem, but it will also maintain your skin's beauty and healthy.

Additionally in addition, it is important to apply a pure oil of black seeds at night prior to sleeping throughout your body. This will nourish your skin, and keep it healthy. If you are suffering from skin disorders such as acne, pimples or eczema, you need to mix one teaspoon of black seed oil and one cup of vinegar, and apply it over the affected locations. Keep this routine going for three or four weeks to get an healthy relief from your acne-related issues.

Furthermore, skin ailments such as Barras are treatable applying black cumin seeds. Simply take 1 teaspoon of black seeds oil and rub it onto the areas affected by it for about the size of a half

an hour prior to going to bed. Use it gently before going to sleep. The next time you get up time, make sure you get a bath and apply gentle soap.

Nigella sativa is the most effective treatment for all types of skin conditions. Particularly, if wrinkles are beginning to appear in your skin, it is recommended to consider applying black cumin seeds and oil, and mixing them together with the right compounds for an ideal skin care solutions.

Minimal Duration: Recommended until the result is satisfactory

HEALTH CONDITION: FOR SNORING

What To Use: Black Seed oil and Lukewarm water

How to Use: Mix 2ml of black cumin (Kalonji) oil into one cup of milk that is lukewarm. Consume it for an hour prior to sleeping each night.

Maximum Duration: Recommended often until snoring stops completely.

HEALTH CONDITION: FOR WEAK EYESIGHT

How to use How to use: Oil extracted from Black Seeds

Method of Use: Apply an ounce of Black Cumin (Kalonji) oil every day in both eyes. It can improve your eyesight.

Minimum Duration Recommend The recommended minimum duration is 7 to 14 days

HEALTH CONDITION: LIBIDO LOSS MALE

What To Use How to Use Original honey

How to Use: Cumin is a powerful ingredient that increases sexual performance and libido. It increases the fertility of males through raising the number of sperm.

Mix honey with Black Cumin powder in equal amounts. Take 1 tablespoon with a full stomach. Do this every day for two weeks.

Minimum Recommended Duration Minimum Duration: 14 days

HEALTH CONDITION: FOR HIV AIDS

What To Use What to Use: Raw Black seeds

What to Take: Drink 2 teaspoons of Black Seed concoction twice daily for six months. (Boil the seeds. It is recommended to drink two spoons daily.

Minimum Term Recommended Minimum Duration: 6 months

HEALTH CONDITION: FOR LEUCODERMA

What To Use What to Use: Raw black seeds powder or milk

What to Take: Consume 1 teaspoon of Black Cumin powder. Let it soak overnight in milk. In the morning, prepare the paste, then spread it on the region affected.

Minimum Time Recommended: Use every day until the result is satisfactory

HEALTH CONDITION: FOR POOR CONCENTRATION

What To Use: Black seed powder, honey

What to do: Use a one half tablespoon of Black Cumin seed powder. Mix it in with Honey. Take it in two doses daily.

Minimum Time Recommended Apply daily until your results are satisfactory

HEALTH CONDITION: FOR MENOPAUSE

How to use The Raw Black Seeds

What to do: Take 2 tablespoons Black Cumin seeds with a cup of water in the morning.

Minimum Duration Recommend Minimum Duration: 7 to 15 Days

HEALTH CONDITION: FOR DIARRHEA

How to use What to Use: Raw Black seeds Null Acacia powder gum

Mix 1 tablespoon of powdered gum from Acacia Nilotic with water. Let the leaves soak in water for one hour. Drink the infusion using a tiny quantities in Black Cumin.

The recommended minimum duration is Between 2 and 5 days

HEALTH CONDITION: FOR RINGWORM

What to use: Vernonia Cinerea, Poppy, Black Cumin seeds, Dry Coconut powder, lukewarm water.

How to use: Make an emulsion of Vernonia Cinerea Poppy, Vernonia Cinerea, black Cumin, dry Coconut powder. Use it for three hours. Rinse it with warm water.

Minimal Duration: Recommended till it has completely cured.

HEALTH CONDITION: FOR GOUT

How to use: Asparagus Racemases, Black Cumin seeds, Fenugreek, Carom

What to Do: Use an equally large amounts of seeds from the listed herb:

Asparagus Racemosus, Black Cumin, Fenugreek and Carom. Consume 5 grams every day in warm water.

The minimum duration recommended is: use till cure.

HEALTH CONDITION: FOR LOWER BACK PAIN

How to use: Asparagus Racemosus, Black Cumin seeds Fenugreek, Carom

Method of Use mix seeds of Asparagus racemosus, black Cumin, Fenugreek and Carom. Consume 1 teaspoon each morning.

Minimal Duration: Recommended until you get good results

Chapter 6: Herbal Treatment For Libido Loss Male 2

What to Take: Consume these herbs: Indian Spider Plant (Safed Muslin India) Liquor Ice (Mulethi from India) 1 tablespoon, trailing Eclipta (Bhringraj in India) 1 tablespoon Velvet Bean (Konch in India) 5 tablespoons, ginger (Adrak in India) : 1.5 tablespoons, Black Henbane (Khurasani Ajavayan in India) 1 tablespoon. Black Cumin (Kala Jeera in India) 2 to 3 teaspoons.

What to do: Mix the two together. Take half a teaspoon of water.

Minimum Recommended Duration: between 2 and 6 weeks.

HEALTH CONDITION: FOR ACNE

What to use Powder of Black Seeds: Kala Jeera powder: 1/2 teaspoon

Basil Tulsi Leaf: crushed 1 teaspoon

Azadirachta Indica: Neem: Leaves: Crushed: 1 teaspoon

Instructions for Apply: Mix all the ingredients. Use on the affected areas for 20 mins. Rinse by rinsing with cool water.

Minimum Time Required: Repeat for 2-5 days

HEALTH CONDITION: FOR ABSCESS

How to use: Black Cumin Powder/seeds, Basil (Tulsi) leaves and Azadirachta Indica (Neem) leaves.

What to Use: Grind the ingredients together. Mix in a little bit of water. Rub it onto the areas affected. Wash with cold water.

Minimum Recommended Duration: Between 2 and 5 days

HEALTH CONDITION: FOR ANTIVIRAL

What to use: 5 grams of Date Palm powder, 8 Ml of Honey and 3ml black cumin seeds oil

What to use: Mix 5 grams Date Palm powder, 8 milliliters of honey and 3 milliliters black cumin seed oil to one cup of hot water. Take 2 teaspoons every day.

Minimum Recommended Duration: between 3 and 6 weeks.

56. HEALTH CONDITION: FOR MEMORY ENHANCER 3

How to Use The best oils to use are: Black Cumin oil

Method of Use: Boil Mint leaves for eight minutes. Include 2ml of Black Cumin oil to it. Keep it in use for one month.

Minimum Recommended Duration: Between 4 and 5 weeks.

HEALTH CONDITION: FOR LEPROSY 4

How to use What to Use: Black Cumin seed oil

Application: Spread Apple juice on the affected area. Massage it gently until it's absorbed by the skin. Following this, apply Black Cumin seed oil for massaging the same region.

Minimum Time Required: Take each day until results are attained.

HEALTH CONDITION: FOR DANDRUFF 16

How to use How to use: Black Cumin Seed oil olive oil, Henna leaves

How to Use: Make a mix made of Black Cumin Seed oil, olive oil, and Henna powder leaves, in 1:3:3 proportions. Warm the mixture. Cool them. Use it to apply on your scalp and hair.

Minimum duration recommended: use every day until the desired result is reached. In most cases, no more than 7 days are required for the best results.

HEALTH CONDITION: FOR FLATULENCE 23

How to use: Use the seeds of black cumin, Peppermint and Fennel

Method of Use: Combine the seeds of black cumin, Peppermint and Fennel in 1:1 ratio. Use it to make tea. It is recommended to drink it at least twice per every day.

The recommended minimum duration is 2-to-5 weeks

HEALTH CONDITION: FOR GALLSTONE FLUSH

What to Use: Black Cumin (Kalonji) oil and Pure Honey

Method of Use: Take an the same amount of black cumin (Kalonji) oil, and honey (She was a honey addict). Mix it all up and put in an e-bottle. Take a teaspoon of the mix with some lukewarm water in empty stomach. Repeat this process regularly until issue is resolved.

The recommended minimum duration is 1 - 2 months.

HEALTH CONDITION: FOR SNORING 1

What To Use What to Use: Raw black seed Golden Bamboo (Baans), Honey

How to Utilize How to Use: Take 2 teaspoons of black cumin (Kalonji) and 2 pieces of dried Golden Bamboo (Baans) leaves. Place them in a glass of water. Boil. Strain. Include one tablespoon of Honey (Shehad). Consume it prior to the bed time.

Minimum Duration: Perform according to the requirements

HEALTH CONDITION: FOR DIABETES 17

What to Use:

Gymnema Sylvestre 50 mg

Dried Bitter Gourd 50 mg

Fenugreek Seeds 50 mg

The black seeds (Black Cumin) 50 mg

Dried Black Plum (Jamun)50 mg

Black Pepper 25 mg

Soy Milk or Butter Milk (Lassi), Water

What to do: Make the finest powder from each herb ingredients and keep in a container

Consume 1/4 teaspoon of the powder with a glass of Soy Milk or Butter Milk (Lassi) in empty stomach.

HEALTH CONDITION: HERBAL TREATMENT FOR DIABETES 19

How to use: Black Cumin seeds (Kalonji) of Kalonji, 6 grams Kasni (chicory) as well as 6 grams of Fenugreek seeds

What to Use: Create an extremely fine powder from 10 grams of black cumin (Kalonji), 6 grams of Kasni (Chicory) and six grams of Fenugreek seeds and keep them in a container. Use 1/3 tsp of this powder, mix it with two drops Nigella seeds oil. Drink the mixture with water every daily.

The minimum duration recommended is every day for at least one month before undergoing a medical checkup.

HEALTH CONDITION: HERBAL TREATMENT FOR DIABETES 22

What to use The Black Cumin is 1 cup of seeds. Add 2/3 cup pomegranate rind and 1/2 Cup of Shahtara (Fumaria Indica)

How to use: Make the powder into a fine paste of 1 cup of black cumin 1 cup of should include seeds. 2/3 cup pomegranate rind and 1/2 1 cup Shahtara (Fumaria Indica)

Then, you can collect it into a vessel. Then, take 1 tsp of the powder, along with 12 drops Black Cumin seeds oil and take it by drinking water in a stomach empty.

The minimum duration recommended is every day for at least one month, and then have a check-up.

HEALTH CONDITION: BLADDER, KIDNEY AND LIVER FUNCTIONS

How to use The oil of black seed as well as other components.

What to do: Both liver and kidney work in regulating the urinary system as well as to eliminate toxins. But, the kidneys are often impacted and is unable to eliminate toxins in those suffering from liver and kidney disease. If you are suffering from liver and kidney issues and liver issues, black seed oil can help speed up the process.

Chapter 7: Allergies Treatments & Prevention

How to use How to use: Black seed oil

How to Use/ Explanations:

The symptoms of allergies like watery eyes sneezing and stuffy nose can cause lots of pain. In particular, if you do not discover a remedy that can be reassembled to eliminate allergy symptoms, it can worsen and causes other severe allergies.

conditions like sinusitis and asthma.

There are a myriad of medicines that treat allergies however most contain a number of adverse consequences. It is therefore best to steer clear of medications that are allopathic and opt for natural remedies like Nigella Sativa oils. The seed of black cumin (Nigella Sativa) has proved to be the ideal remedy for a variety of allergic conditions. Black cumin seed oil is an antihistamine that reduces common signs of allergy, like watery eyes, sneezing and so on. Black seeds also helps to reduce allergic reactions that happen during the winter months.

The reason you're suggested to utilize the black seed oil to lessen allergic symptoms is that it acts as an bronchodilator as well. The bronchi-dilating properties of Nigella Sativa reduce the size of bronchis and the bronchioles. Additionally, it reduces resistance to air in the respiratory tract and improves the circulation of air through the lung. Due to this dilation allergies and asthma issues are more unlikely to develop.

But, it's essential to know how to utilize black cumin seeds to treat allergy issues as well as gaining the advantages of antihistamines and an effect on broncodilating. Do not to use

Black cumin seeds that are solid and black to treat your allergic reactions. This could cause adverse negative effects.

Always apply black cumin oil to help treat allergies. Here's how to make use of black seed oil in treatment of allergies:

If symptoms of allergy begin appearing, only take a teaspoon black cumin oil every each day. If you use this oil for a 2 weeks or so, and you'll be rid of the symptoms soon.

If your allergic reaction is now a chronic asthma, respiratory or bronchial difficulty, then combine a teaspoon black cumin oil with coffee. The mixture should be taken every day before waking up or sleeping time.

Furthermore, it is recommended to apply and rub the black seed oil over the sensitive areas in your body. This will help eliminate the cause.

Therefore, you should follow the easy steps that, if implemented and follow, you can say goodbye to allergy-related issues for ever.

HEALTH CONDITION: FOR DEBILITY

What To Use: Black Seed oil Original Honey

Method of Use Mix 1 teaspoon Honey along with 2 drops of black cumin seed oil twice a daily.

The recommended minimum duration is between 3 and 6 weeks.

HEALTH CONDITION: FOR SCARS, SUNBURN, MARKS

How to use How to use: Black seed oil

How to Use: Cumin Seed Oil is rich in Thymoquinone as well as Vitamin A. These vitamins aid in the regeneration of skin cells. They also makes the skin more supple. This helps fade the appearance of spots and burn spots.

Use 1 to 2 teaspoons of black cumin seed Oil. Place it directly on the area affected. Apply a gentle massage for between 5 and 10 minutes. Repeat the massage twice a throughout the month for one month in order to remove burned marks.

The minimum recommended duration is 4 weeks

HEALTH CONDITION: FOR CARBUNCLE.

Carbuncle is a skin disease. the Skin.

The bacterial disease that triggers an accumulation of Boils are known as Carbuncle. The cause is the Staphylococcus Aureus bacteria, which is a bacterial infection that affects the lower Skin. The bacteria attack a set of hair Follicles. This causes swelling that causes Boils. There are multiple Boils which are affecting the Subcutaneous Tissues. It creates a lump, and has pus underneath the skin. It's typically found in the Throat, Nose, Thighs back Hips and Neck. The bacteria can infect

A group of hair Follicles. It is called Carbuncle. If it is infected by a single Hair follicle it's called Furuncle.

How to use How to use: Black seed oil

What to do Make a mixture of half teaspoon Black Cumin Seed Oil in one glass of water that is lukewarm. Take it two times a day.

The minimum duration recommended: use until you have achieved the goal.

HEALTH CONDITION: FOR COUGH

How to use: Black seeds oil, ginger

Method of Use Apply Black Cumin Seed Oil on your chest prior to getting ready to go to go to bed. Wrap your body in a towel after applying the oil.

OR Make a mixture of one teaspoon Black Cumin Seed Oil in one cup of Ginger tea. Take it in two doses throughout the day.

The recommended minimum duration is 2-to-7 days

HEALTH CONDITION: FOR OSTEOPOROSIS

(a medical issue in which the bones break down and become delicate due to loss of bone tissue usually due to hormonal changes or deficiencies in vitamin D.)

What to Use: Babchi Oil, Black Cumin Oil, Birch Oil Sesame Oil

What to Mix How to Use: Mix 5 drops of Babchi Oil, 2 drops of Black Cumin Oil, 2 drops of Birch Oil and 2 teaspoons of Sesame Oil. Apply a gentle massage to the area affected.

The minimum duration recommended is for a minimum of two weeks.

HEALTH CONDITION: RELIEVES INSECT BITES

How to use What to Use: Oil from black seeds

What to use: In case you've recently been bitten by mosquitoes or other insect using black seed oil onto the area affected can ease pain and itching instantly. This is among the more popular applications of the oil of black seeds, and is considered to be one of the top solutions for treating insect bites naturally.

Minimum Duration Recommend: Apply when needed.

HEALTH CONDITION: FOR MENINGITIS

What to Use: Black Seeds oil

What to use the Potency: This amazing herb has been proven beneficial in the management of the meningitis. Certain studies have proven that it's among the most effective natural cures in the field of treatment today. Just take 1 teaspoon each day for relief.

The minimum duration recommended is to consume 1-2 teaspoons of the drug daily to get relief.

HEALTH CONDITION: FOR HEALTHY BONE MARROW GROWTH

What is the best way to use it What to Use: Oil from black seeds

The best way to use it The research has proven that black extract of seeds to boost bone marrow cells' development rate by a staggering 150 percent. According to a variety of research studies that were conducted on a variety of subjects. It's more impressive it has been proven to slow the growth rate of all cancers by a minimum of 50 percent.

The minimum recommended dosage is 1 to 2 spoons a day until the time you need it.

HEALTH CONDITION: NATURAL REMEDY FOR COLIC (FOR BABIES)

How to Use: Black seed oil Honey, lemon, black seed oil

What to use: If you have a child suffering with colic is an extremely difficult time for you and your family. While the reason for colic remains a mystery however, it is known the fact that black seed oil has been shown to be a treatment for colic that is natural. It's best to start in small doses and build up slowly. In this scenario would be to prepare a cup of tea made from lemon, honey as well as a couple of (3-5) drop of oil from black seeds. Then, give the baby one baby spoon every day.

Chapter 8: Repairs Prostate Problems

How to use How to use: Oil extracted from Black Seeds

What to use: Prostate health is a major issue for many people around the world and figuring out healthy methods to enhance it is stressful. The good news is that black seed oil has been utilized for centuries in order to manage and enhance prostate health. Research has proven it can aid in the fight against prostate cancer. Take 2 spoons daily.

Recommended Minimum Duration: 1-to-3 months

HEALTH CONDITION: GENERAL WEAKNESS (LETHARGY)

How to use How to use: Black seed oil

What to use: A lot of us suffer from depressions and emotional lows throughout our lives along with physical one. If you want to boost your spirits health, energy and general wellbeing it is hard to beat the black seed oil. It's among the most effective herbal remedies that can improve your the overall health of a person both physical and mental. Take 2 spoons daily.

The recommended minimum duration is 1-to-3 months

HEALTH CONDITION: FOR HYPER-SALIVATION

How to use What to Use: Black Seed Oil, ginger juice

How to Use: Crush fresh ginger. Extract the juice. Mix 2 tablespoons of oil from black seeds with 1 teaspoon of ginger juice. Gargle your mouth with the mixture, keep it in place and let it circulate through your saliva glands, as well as the entire mouth. Do this for 7-20 minutes. Then, spit them out. Mix 1 spoon of black seed oil and half the ginger juice. Take this drink. Do this every day. While sleeping you should also sleep with your back in order to accelerate the process of improvement.

Minimum Term is 7-14 days to get a complete cure.

HEALTH CONDITION: DEEP CLEANS PORES

The Best Uses Oil from Back Seeds

What to use: The result of having a weak immunity is the formation of excessive sebum, which can clog the pores of your skin. Take a small amount orally and rub on the affected area after taking the shower to get best outcomes. It will show the improvement immediately, and your pores should be completely clear after 2 weeks of consistent usage.

The minimum recommended duration is Two weeks.

HEALTH CONDITION: - TREATS SCHIZOPHRENIA

How to use What to Use: Oil from black seeds

The Best Method to Use While it isn't the case that both are not the least of them, thymoquinone found in the black cumin seed oil extract can be beneficial in decreasing inflammation as well as helping to treat schizophrenia. There has been research that shows improvements for patients who've taken the black seed oil for a natural treatment in comparison to patients who didn't.

Minimum Time Optimal: Take regularly 2 tablespoons of water daily until you notice a significant improvements.

Oil from black seeds is a great remedy for hair

HEALTH CONDITION: FOR SCALP MASSAGE, HAIR GLOW, HAIR SOFTENING ETC

What To Use What to Use: Black Seed Oil, olive oil

What to do Regular scalp massages is a great method to increase circulation to your scalp. This will in turn encourage healthy hair development. Some curlies make use of this routine to ease stress for their hair curly routine. If you want to use black seeds for your next scalp massage, you can try applying 1 teaspoon of black seed oil two tablespoons of olive oil (or an oil carrier that you prefer) thoroughly on your scalp to stimulate hair to grow. Afterward, rinse with an exfoliating conditioner.

Recommended Minimum Duration: Us frequently as often as you need.

HEALTH CONDITION: HAIR LOSS REMEDY

How to use for: Black seeds, extra olive oil that is virgin,

How to Use:

1.Add 2 tablespoons of seeds from black cumin into 5 cups of water.

2.Boil at a simmer for about 10 mins. Then let it cool.

3.Strain to remove the seeds.

4.Pour the black cumin solution into an ice container.

5.Add 1 tablespoon extra-virgin olive oil.

6.Massage this mix on your scalp, at least two times each week.

7.Let it sit on your hair for between 30 and 1 hour. Then, wash your hair.

8.Keep the mix in the fridge for two weeks max (without the addition of preservatives).

Minimum Time Optimum Utilize as needed.

Continue reading to discover what black seed oil can do to provide your hair with a an instant glow and also how you can incorporate it in your daily hair care routine.

BENEFITS OF BLACK SEED OIL FOR HAIR 1. Hydrates and Nourishes the Hair

Do you want silky, hydrated and hair that is smooth and silky (yes you can!)? A certified trichologist and a creative colorist Bridgette Hill suggests that Black seed oil is thought to nourish, moisturize and smooth hair. But, she adds that an important caveat, just like other herbs and remedies is that the results are mostly based on anecdotes and not supported by evidence. So you'll need to give this a shot yourself to check out how it affects your hair.

2. It helps with Scalp Condition

If you're suffering from scalp or skin problems If you're suffering from skin issues or scalp problems, the oil of black seeds could assist with this. "Due to its anti-bacterial and anti-fungal properties, [black seed oil] can help resolve skin imbalances such as eczema and psoriasis on the scalp and body," states Jenelle Kim DACM, LAc, creator and formulator of JBK Wellness Labs. Certain studies have proven that oil extracted from black seeds could assist in the treatment and management of issues with scalp that are better than comparable to prescribed medications.

3. Can Keep Dandruff at Bay

If you're suffering from Dandruff, read this. "Basic science studies have demonstrated that extracts of black seed oil can help decrease the growth of various fungal organisms" thanks to its antibacterial it's anti-inflammatory, anti-fungal, and anti-bacterial qualities, claims Sandy Skotnicki, MD, an expert dermatologist who is board certified as well as the creator of Beyond Soap. "Normal naturally occurring fungus species in the hair are believed as a factor in the formation of dandruff. The evidence supports the use of black seed oil in conjunction with other ingredients that deliver nutrients for reducing dandruff" Dr. Skotnicki asserts. However, it's not any clinical studies to support the claims, but the evidence from anecdotes is in support.

Chapter 9: How To Use Black Seed Oil For Hair

1. Use A Hair Product That Contains Black Seed Oil

One of the easiest ways to test the black seed oil's effects for your hair is to include the product for your hair in your routine that has the oil. This could be shampoos, serums for hair as well as hair masks. Dr. Skotnicki recommends checking the content that the oil's extract has. "Look for at least 0.5 percent Nigella sativa, which was used in the study and showed good hair growth," she advises. Dr. Skotnicki notes that during the study, the oils were applied to the hair using an oil that had 0.5 percent Nigella in sativa each day for three months. That is why consistency across a time time will yield the most effective results.

2. Make A DIY Hair Treatment

For your personal treatment using black seed oil at home, consult Dr. Kim says to mix the oil in with a different carrier oil like coconut, olive, or castor oil in order to enhance the effectiveness of the oil. Hill's preferred method is to use oils such as black seed oil for an anti-shampoo treatment to your hair and scalp. Apply the treatment on hair that isn't washed "Allow the oil to process for a minimum of 30 minutes," Hill states. To achieve the best results, Hill recommends sleeping wearing the treatment in the hair. Make sure you use the right pillowcase, one that you won't like getting oily.

HEALTH CONDITION: PREVENTS MUSCLE CRAMPS AND SPASMS -

What to Use: Black Seed oil

What to do: The antispasmodic as well as anti-inflammatory components present in the oil of black seeds make it extremely effective in stopping as well as easing muscle cramps/spasms. It can be consumed in a liquid form or rub it onto the areas affected and see results in a matter of minutes. It is also recommended to take it in a pill and apply it to the external area.

The minimum duration recommended is until the desired result is reached. Continue using until you have achieved the result.

HEALTH CONDITION: KILLS LEUKEMIA CELLS -

How to use What to Use: Oil from black seeds

The best way to use it: A study revealed that black seeds have beneficial effects against the proliferation of the human myeloblastic leukemia cells HL-60. The reason for this can be traced back to thymoquinone in it that makes it a potent cure. Two spoons of it each day.

The recommended minimum duration is 1-to-3 months

HEALTH CONDITION: SUPPRESSES BREAST CANCER

How to use How to use: Black seed oil

The best way to use it: The oil of black seed showed constant ability to inhibit the proliferation of breast cancer cells in the long term treatment. The research showed that greater dosages led to more effective reduction. Start with one spoon in the morning and one spoon in the evening (2 spoons per day) in the beginning month. After the second month, consume 3 spoons a day (1 spoon in the morning and afternoon; 1 spoon evening one spoon evening, and the other at evening).

The recommended minimum duration is between 2 and 6 months.

HEALTH CONDITION: RELIEVES TONSIL INFLAMMATION (ACUTE TONSILLOPHARYNGITIS)

How to Use What to Use: Black Seed Oil, Honey

What to use: Reduces Tonsil inflammation (Acute Tonsillopharyngitis) Black seeds have been shown to ease the pain in their throats caused by inflammation of tonsils. They also reduce the necessity for painkillers. Research has proven it to be one of the most efficient home remedies to treat throat pain. It's also an excellent alternative to treating sore throats. Mix 20ml with 5ml of honey. Take 2 spoons daily.

Minimum Time Recommended: Use until the desired result is reached.

HEALTH CONDITION: EFFICIENT MRSA TREATMENT

What to Use:

What to use: Methicillin resistance Staphylococcus aureus (MSRA) has affected healthcare facilities and hospitals across the globe as staph-related infections become ever more intolerant to antibiotics that are generic. It is caused by the weakening of the immune system black seeds can cause MSRA.

It is a fantastic alternative to many of the antibiotics available today. There are many infections which black seeds have been well-known to cure most likely this one of the top one.

The most troublesome for seniors (since the procedure is required in certain instances), MSRA can be caused by a variety of inexplicably high discomfort throughout the body. However, studies have shown that it is not a cause for concern.

The research has shown the black seed oil compound are a powerful way to stop the spread of MRSA and eliminate MRSA completely.

Minimum duration recommended: consume 2 spoons daily, until the results are seen.

HEALTH CONDITION: TREATS EARACHES

How to use How to Use olive oil

What to use: The black seed oil, mixed with olive oil (1/2 teaspoon each) which is heated and then dripped into the ear that is affected an effective way to get instant relief from ear pain. Place an ear cover or a scarf on the affected ear following dripping for 2 minutes before letting it dry.

Maximum Duration: The results appear to be faster. Apply for one to three days for a full treatment.

Health Condition:

What to Use:

How to Use:

Minimum Duration Recommended:

Health Condition: For Chest Congestion

What to use What to Use: Black Seed Oil, Honey

Method of Use: Rub the oil with black seeds on your chest in order to rid your body of congestion and accumulation. The oil will do wonders when combined with honey. It is also possible to chew them too.

Minimum Recommended Duration is 7-15 days.

Health Condition: Improves Memory (Dementia) -

What is the best way to use it What to Use: Oil from black seeds

What to use The results of research have shown that consumption of black seeds improves the memory, cognition as well as your attention. Recent research has shown that it can boost your memory and improve memory retention, both long and short-term. Use 1 spoon every both at dawn and evening.

Minimum Duration: Recommended every day as needed.

Health Condition: Treats Moles

The Best Uses back seed oil

What to use How to Use well-known benefits for skin is oils from black seeds, they aid to eliminate moles through repressing their development and clearing the skin. Massage the oil onto those areas that are affected.

Minimal Duration Recommend Utilize as needed

Health Condition: Relieves Insect Bites

How to Use What to Use: Oil from black seeds

The best way to use it: If you've been recently bit by mosquitoes or other bugs using black seed oil to the area affected helps alleviate itchiness and pain instantly. This is among the most commonly used uses of black seed oil which is considered to be one of the top natural cures for bites from insects.

Chapter 10: Lowers Anxiety, Stress And Depression

How to Use What to Use: Black Seed/Powder, Ashwagandha, Chamomile

What to use What to do: We have learned that inflammation causes negative effects on psychosis as well as mental health issues. The results of studies have proven that the oil of black seeds to be much more effective at maintaining your mood and lower anxiety levels following daily usage for thirty days. Many advocate anti-inflammatory therapy in lieu of antidepressant medications to help ease anxiety. Combine all the ingredients in 5:2:2 proportion. Make tea. Do not add sugar or milk. Mix and drink when warm or cool. Consume half of a glass every day.

Minimum Duration As long as is needed. The minimum is usually 14 days.

HEALTH CONDITION: PREVENTS ANEMIA

How to use How to use: Black seed oil

The best way to use it: Many of us suffer from the risk from blood thinning (anemia) as it could put our body and our health at risk. Black seeds are there to help as they've proven to treat and prevent anemia and eliminate it in a variety of cases and research. A spoon of black seeds in the early morning and at night can help tremendously.

Minimal Duration use as required.

HEALTH CONDITION: TREATS OBESITY

How to use How to use: Black seed oil

The best way to utilize it is that the majority of people who are obese have an the increased risk of developing the immune system as well as cancer, insulin resistance as well as cardiovascular ailments and cancer, the black seed oil can be the perfect natural solution for treating. It's been proven to have antioxidant properties that have been proven in many studies carried out by researchers across the globe. A teaspoon of it every in the morning and at night can help a lot assist.

Minimum Recommended Duration: between 1 and 3 months.

HEALTH CONDITION: DETOXIFIES BODY -

How to use: Black seed oil

What to use Toxicity: It is a huge issue for many people, so finding a method to reduce it may appear impossible. It is good to know that the black seed oil has been utilized to detoxify for a long time, and scientific studies show that it reduces toxic levels in the body in a significant way. Use 1 spoon in the each day and at night.

The recommended minimum duration is between 1 and 4 weeks.

HEALTH CONDITION: TREATS LYMPHOMA -

How to use What to Use: Oil extracted from black seeds

What to use: Lymphatic cancer (another name for Lymphoma) is a very painful illness that is affecting millions of people around the world. Numerous studies have been conducted showing that black seed extract is powerful in the elimination of lymphatic cancerous cells. The research suggests taking daily doses (1-2 teaspoons) to get the best outcomes. Making 2 teaspoons daily of blackseed oil goes way to aiding in

The recommended minimum duration is between 2 and 3 months.

HEALTH CONDITION: FOR HEART ATTACK

What to use What to Use: Black Sed oil, goat milk

How to Use: Mix 4 ml black cumin seed oil into one cup of Goat Milk. Take it two times a day for a week. Then, you can do it twice each per day.

The recommended minimum duration is 2-to-3 months

Chapter 11: Getting Started With Black Seed

The author will deal with two different intriguing Indian and Middle-Eastern spices, which are commonly called "black seed" due to the resemblance of their flavors. This can be a confusing subject because both of these ingredients are very different (with distinct flavor) and come from diverse sources and they are often referred to interchangeably. When I was researching this cookbook I finally decided it would be best to mix the two Kalonji (nigella sativa) and Black Cumin (bunium bulbocastanum, also known as Black Jeera) and in order to make a recipe list that makes the most from "black seed" in all its beauty.

As you are making your food with these ingredients, make note that a recipe may require black cumin seeds or Sativa seeds. Nigella is a seed that has a sweet onion flavor that is nutty and nutty is a fantastic replacement for sesame or poppy seeds. Nigella can be used in everything from salads pastas, potato dishes and baked items. Nigella sativa provides a distinct blend of flavors.

Note that nigella sativa typically comes in various varieties. The most popular, which you will find in many grocery stores that sell health foods includes Black seed oil. It can be utilized widely in this recipe or in the everyday cooking routine.

The black cumin flavor isn't like nigella Sativa. It's a smokey, semi-sweet taste. Therefore, it's more suited to salads and baked goods. However, it's ideal for large meals for example, curried foods as well as soups, sauces for instance. It's a very popular spice across India however it seldom encountered on the menus of the West (much as nigella sativa is actually).

A few other terms for the species can be:

Roman coriander

Black sesame

Black caraway

Health Effects of Middle-Eastern Black Seed

The prophet Mohammed once stated "black seed can cure everything but death" (likely in reference to the nigella sativa). Recently, black seed has been gaining popularity within the world of health food as a new marvel ingredient that is capable of nearly anything, minus applying it to stumps to help grow an limb missing.

According to a database created by Green Med Info [1], black seeds have been associated to healing properties for treating diseases such as

Chronic chronic

Infections caused by bacteria

Ulcers

Asthma

Blood pressure that is high

Inflammatory-related illnesses

Fungal infections

Hypertension

Spasms

Infections caused by viruses

Diabetes

Liver disorders

Kidney disease

and cancers of all kinds

As for its health benefits the black seed has been extensively studied because of its capability to fight the spread of bacterial infections. That includes resistance to antibacterial "superbugs" now plaguing hospitals all over the world. The black seed is also promising against fungi and viruses.

The health benefits are related to three substances that are found in black seeds three of them: thymoquinone, thymohydr and the chemical thymol. These three chemicals work together to fight diseases and help the body eliminate pathogens. In combination with the anti-inflammatory benefits you can see the black seed as the perfect cocktail to fight off disease.

The benefits of black seeds include an Croatian study, which looked into the properties that fight tumors of two chemicals which showed positive outcomes[2[2. The study looked into the Black seed oil's effects on regenerative processes on liver function[3], research in the antiidiabetic qualities of the black seed[4as well as a myriad of studies on its anti-microbial benefits.

According to this research It is clear that this black seed is the most powerful superfood and is a crucial component for people who suffers from illnesses that can be helped by a healthy diet.

Making Black Seed Curry

It is possible to find a variety of supplements made from black seeds at the health stores, however I would rather get it by cooking using the spice. Black cumin as well as Nigeria sativa are readily available all over every online store such as Amazon. They can be added to nearly anything comparable seeds such as sesame could taste great on. Moreover, it's recommended that you roast the nigella sativa seeds in a skillet using a little oil prior to preparing the menu.

In this book, there are a lot of Middle Eastern and Indian inspired recipes that you can try. The recipes I have included are closely with the history of black seeds because it's been utilized throughout the ages. These include eggplant-based dishes that include hummus or chickpeas curried dishes as well as stews and soups pilafs and many baked items where Nigeria sativa is used like when you use sesame or poppy seeds.

It is interesting to note that this may be the sole black seed cookbook I've come across. Although the spice is as old as it is however, its popularity among the West is still a distant memory. It was only in these past few months that it started to make waves on the scene, and I'm sure it's likely to be seeing a greater amount of it very soon.

You're probably eager to start. We'll dive right into recipe!

Appetizers

Spicy Chickpeas stuffed with tomatoes, spicy chickpeas, as well as Spinach

The blend of flavors that make up this dish, as well as its healthy qualities is a fantastic method to start using black seeds.

Servings: 4

INGREDIENTS

1 tablespoon vegetable oil

1/2 tsp black seeds (nigella sativa)

1 1/2 tsp fennel seeds

1 large onion chopped

400g chopped tomatoes in a can.

3 green chillies seeded and cut in chunks lengthways

3-4 tsp light brown sugar

1 teaspoon paprika

1 teaspoon turmeric

1/2 teaspoon black cumin

410g of chickpeas in a can, cleaned and draining

1 tbsp tamarind

1 Tbsp fresh chopped coriander

120 g baby spinach leaves

DIRECTIONS

Pour the oil into an enormous skillet, and place on medium-low heat. In the skillet, add the black and fennel seeds. Fry for around 15 minutes.

Incorporate the chopped onion, and cook for about 5-7 minutes over moderate heat, until it becomes golden and transparent.

Mix in chillies, chickpeas and sugar. Add paprika, paprika, black cumin, and turmeric and then bring the mixture to a boil.

Reduce the heat to a simmer and let it cook for 10 minutes.

Include the tamarind, coriander and spinach leaves, Stir and cook for a few minutes until the spinach leaves are tender.

Chicken Vegetable Salad served with Avocado Pesto

Healthy, high-fiber and nutritious salad that includes beetroots, broccoli, chicken breasts, and pesto made of garlic and avocado. Nigella Sativa seeds give the perfect kick of flavor. Pesto in itself is a gourmet. Watercress is also a great complement to the chicken. You can make extra pesto to use in various meals. THIS RECIPE IS SERIOUSLY GOOD.

Servings: 4

INGREDIENTS

250g broccoli, stemmed

2 teaspoons grape seed oil

3 skinless, chicken breasts

1 onion red finely cut

100g bag of watercress

2 beetroots raw (about 175g) Peeled, julienned and peeled or grated

1 TSP black seeds

The avocado pesto is the basis for this recipe.

Small package of basil

1 avocado

1/2 cloves of garlic, crushed

The walnuts are 25g in size broken into pieces

1 Tbsp of the oil of rapeseed

1. 1 Lemon juice, and the rind

DIRECTIONS

Slice the broccoli into florets. put them in a pot filled with boiling water. Cook for about 3 minutes. Transfer to a colander. clean under cold running water.

1. Heat half a teaspoon of grape seed oil into a large skillet. Then add the broccoli, and cook for two minutes on each the side, until it is golden brown. Then, remove the broccoli from the skillet and allow it to rest for 5 minutes before letting it cool.

In the same skillet, cook the chicken until it is brown on both sides for around 3 minutes each. Transfer the chicken to a plate, and let it sit for a few minutes to cool. Shred the shredded pieces into small chunks.

Save 3-4 basil leaves to garnish. Put the remainder in a blender, along with avocados, walnuts garlic, olive oil, 2 tbsp of cold water, along with 1 teaspoon lemon juice. Sprinkle with salt and black pepper, and blend until it is smooth.

In a bowl add the onions to lemon juice. Let it rest for about a minute.

The watercress should be placed on the large plate. Add the broccoli and onions. Followed by the chicken and beetroot pieces.

Sprinkle the lemon rind and black seeds Add basil leaves. Serve alongside the avocado pesto you've prepared.

Carrot and Fennel Salad

Servings: 6

INGREDIENTS

2 large carrots chopped into sticks thin or grated

2 large fennel bulbs cut in quarters and thinly slice

1. 1/3 cup cashew nuts broken into pieces

Juice 1 lemon

2 tbsp olive oil

1 teaspoon mustard seed

1 tsp nigella seeds

DIRECTIONS

Cut the fennel into pieces and then place it in a bowl, along with carrots that have been grated.

Heat a pan on low heat. Incorporate the nuts, and cook for about 3-4 mins until fragrant and golden. Then remove the skillet from the heat and let cool. Serve the cooked vegetables.

The same pan cook the oil, and then cook the black and mustard seeds approximately a minute. Then add the lemon juice, and mix thoroughly.

Pour the mix over the salad, then toss until it is all mixed.

Chapter 12: White Radish Salad

Try this easy and tasty salad that is packed with nutritious vegetables and spice.

Servings: 4

INGREDIENTS

1 huge Indian white radish, grated

Salt and Pepper

2 tbsp vinegar

a large amount of sugar

2 tablespoons olive oil

1/8 tsp black seeds

1 1/2 tsp cumin seeds

1/2 tsp black mustard seeds

DIRECTIONS

Crumble the radish and place it in an ice-cold bowl. Mix in the vinegar, sugar add some salt, pepper and.

Add the oil in a small saucepan and cook on medium. In the same skillet, add cumin and black seeds, and cook for about 3 to 4 minutes. As they begin to melt, pour the olive oil and seeds on top of the salad. Toss it for a good coating.

Enjoy.

Spicy Rice Pilaf

The dark-colored pilaf made up of nigella Sativa as well as black cumin. Additional healthy ingredients like cinnamon, cilantro, and more make this a nutritional powerhouse recipe. Take this food every day and stay healthy to the age of 120 (if you're willing to live for long enough to witness society replaced by robots).

Servings: 8

INGREDIENTS

2 tablespoons coconut oil or olive oil

1 large onion minced finely

2 cloves

3 cardamom pods, crushed

1 cinnamon stick split into 3 pieces

1/2 teaspoon of black cumin seeds

1/2 teaspoon nigella seeds

3 tbsp fresh cilantro leaves, chopped

4 cups chicken broth

1/2 cup chopped almonds to toast, as garnish

2 1/2 cups basmati rice

DIRECTIONS

The oil should be poured in an enormous saucepan, and then heat to medium-high heat.

Include the onions, the cardamom pods cumin seeds, cloves, cinnamon stick, black seeds and simmer for approximately 7-10 minutes. Stir frequently.

Add the rice and cook for about a minute, then add the chicken broth and bring to a simmer.

Reduce the temperature to a simmer and allow it to simmer for 20 mins, with the lid on. Take off the lid, then place the pot in an absorbent towel, and then put the lid on. Allow the rice to remain for at least 20 minutes.

Fluff the rice using an fork prior to serving. serve it with almonds and chopped cilantro.

Eggplants in a Spicy Sauce

Eggplants are an essential ingredient in The Middle Eastern regions where nigella isativa as well as black cumin come from.

Servings: 4-6

INGREDIENTS

4 tablespoons olive or canola oil

1/8 teaspoon ground asafetida

1/2 tsp of skinned yellow split peas

1/2 teaspoon whole mustard seeds

1/2 teaspoon whole black or cumin seeds

1/2 teaspoon whole Nigerian seeds

1/2 tsp whole seed fennel

One medium onion chopped

2 cloves of garlic cut

600-700 g Italian eggplants, cut

Two medium-sized tomatoes grated

1 1/4-1/2 teaspoons cayenne pepper

1 cup of chicken stock, or water

1 teaspoon of salt

DIRECTIONS

Add olive oil in a pan that is set on a stove with a moderate heat. Then add the split peas, and cook until brown.

Mix in the nigella seeds mustard seeds, fennel seeds as well as cumin. Cook for 30 seconds.

Add the onions, and simmer for around 1-2 minutes. When the onions begin to turn dark Add the eggplant and garlic.

Cook for approximately five minutes. Mix in the tomatoes. simmer for another five minutes, after that, add the liquid or stock. Sprinkle with salt and black pepper, and bring the dish to a simmer.

Reduce the heat until it is low, and then let it simmer for 20 mins, until the eggplants have softened while stirring frequently.

Take a break from the heat and relax.

Crispy Fried Potatoes

Simply follow a few easy steps, and these delicious potatoes can be cooked and served.

Servings: 6-8

INGREDIENTS

13 cup olive oil (divided)

1 cup black seeds

1 teaspoon sea salt

Sea salt that is flaky

1kg large sweet potatoes

DIRECTIONS

Peel the potatoes, then cut them into cubes. Sprinkle with sea salt.

Add 1 teaspoon olive oil to an enormous non-stick pan and place it over a moderate-high temperature. Incorporate the potatoes then gently mix with a the spatula of plastic to cover.

Place the lid on and cook on low heat for 20-25 mins while stirring often until they have a an golden crust, and become soft in the middle.

While you fry the potatoes Toast the black seeds in a large skillet on moderate heat, stirring frequently until they are fragrant and lightly golden.

Arrange the cooked potatoes in a serving dish and sprinkle them with the toasted seeds and sea salt flaky, drizzle the rest of the oil, and then serve.

Quick and Easy Tomato Relish

The Indian spice can be used as an accompaniment to the main course, served on rice, or alongside crispy pita chips. It's also a recipe from the past which makes use of nigella sativa.

Servings: 2

INGREDIENTS

1 tiny red onion

2 tomatoes cut

1 chili very finely chopped

Fresh coriander leaves

Juice 1 lemon

1 TSP salt

1/2 teaspoon garam masala

1 tsp nigella seeds

DIRECTIONS

Finely chop chillies, onions and tomatoes and put them in smaller bowl.

Add chopped coriander. Sprinkle it with salt the nigella seeds, garam masala. Drizzle it with lemon juice freshly squeezed and mix well.

Serve with potatoes fried and pilaf.

Flavorful Sauteed Green Beans

This tasty appetizer is loaded with proteins and delicious flavors. There are many beans that you'd like. It's also great that it will take just a little time to cook it.

Servings: 6

INGREDIENTS

900 g green beans, trimmed, cut

3/4 cup coconut that is unsweetened and shredded

1 1/2 tsp of kosher salt

1 teaspoon black seeds

1/4 cup of canola oil

1 Tbsp yellow mustard seeds

24 leaves of curry broken

DIRECTIONS

Add the oil to the large pan of frying set over a medium heat.

When the mixture is hot Add the mustard seeds as well as black seeds. Saute for around 1 minute until the seeds are fragrant. Then add the curry leaves, and continue to saute for a further minute.

Chapter 13: Moroccan Chickpea Patties

The spicy chickpea patties be a delight to your taste. You must have the right ingredients on the ready and prepare for this unique dessert.

Servings: 8

INGREDIENTS

One small onion chopped

2-3 cloves garlic, peeled

1 cup vegetable oil and some oil for cooking

1 can of chickpeas washed and draining (or 1-1.5 cups of cooked)

1 lemon juiced

1/4 cup chickpeas or oatmeal flour and 2 tablespoons to coat

2 tablespoons parsley

1 teaspoon of black seeds

1/4 teaspoon of cinnamon

1 teaspoon of salt

1 teaspoon ground coriander

1/4 teaspoon cayenne

1. 1/4 teaspoon black pepper

1 teaspoon of ground ginger

DIRECTIONS

Heat olive oil inside a frying pan, and then set it over moderate-high heat.

Add garlic and onions and cook until the onions turn translucent and golden, around 4 minutes.

Add the chickpeas in the microwave safe bowl, and cook for 2 minutes on high until they are heated to the desired temperature.

Puree the warm chickpeas, onions cooked and chickpea flour Parsley lemon juice cinnamon, cumin and cayenne ginger, coriander as well as black pepper into the blender.

Form the mix into patties. Then cover them in flour.

Add a couple of tablespoons of oil into an oven-proof skillet large enough for cooking and place it over a medium temperature.

The patties should be placed in the hot oil, and cook approximately 3 minutes on each the side, until the patties develop a the golden crust.

Enjoy

Baked Asparagus with black seeds

It's a nutritious and delicious dish to serve with a side of rice and it is easy to put together.

Servings: 4-6

INGREDIENTS

450 grams of asparagus

1. 1/2 teaspoons olive oil

1 teaspoon of salt

Taste of pepper

1 teaspoon of black seeds

DIRECTIONS

Heat oven until 220°C.

Remove the woody end of the root on the spears of asparagus. Slightly remove the lower section of the spears. Then rinse them under cold water. The asparagus should be rinsed and placed on a baking tray covered with aluminum foil.

Sprinkle with salt, then drizzle olive oil over the top. In the oven, roast for about 10 to 12 minutes, or until the desired degree of doneness.

In a pan, toast the black seeds on moderate heat for several minutes, until they become fragrant.

Remove the asparagus from the oven. Sprinkle with seeds of black and serve.

Persian Chickpea Salad

Servings: 4-6

INGREDIENTS

1 can of chickpeas drain

2 tbsp olive oil

1 TSP seeds

1 clove of garlic, cut

1 1/2 2 tbsp grated ginger

1 lime juiced

1 tomato, diced

1/2 cup of cilantro chopped

1/2 cup of parsley chopped

Salt, peppers according to your preference

DIRECTIONS

Add the chickpeas tomatoes, garlic black seeds, the chopped herb, ginger as well as olive oil in a bowl for salad.

Add salt and pepper, then mix well. Enjoy.

Simple Cabbage Salad

Cilantro as well as black seeds together with fresh thyme leaves as well as lemon juice makes this easy salad nutritious and tasty.

Servings: 6

INGREDIENTS:

1 medium fennel bulb, stemmed

1 large (900g) Head of cabbage

1/3 cup olive oil

2 tablespoons freshly squeezed juice of a lemon

3TBS of red vinegar wine

1/4 cup of fresh Thyme leaves

1 teaspoon salt

1/2 teaspoon freshly ground pepper

2 tsp mustard powder

2 tsp fennel seeds

2 tsp cilantro seeds

DIRECTIONS

The core should be removed from the cabbage. Slice the cabbage thinly as well as the fennel bulb, and then place into a large salad bowl. By using your fingers to break the cabbage into fine strips. Set aside.

Crush the cilantro and black seeds seeds with a pestle and mortar until they are finely crushed. Transfer the mixture to a bowl.

Add mustard powder fresh squeezed lemon juice, and olive oil. Combine well.

Then add the mix to the chopped cabbage and fennel Then add the thyme leaves. stir well to mix. The salad should sit for five to ten minutes prior to serving.

Chapter 14: Rice And Black Beans

The recipe may seem simple and has a straightforward name, but the flavor is quite unique. Cumin, black seed garlic and cayenne create an aroma that you must taste to yourself.

About 3 servings per meal.

INGREDIENTS

White rice 34 cup raw and uncooked

1 tsp olive oil

400 ml vegetable broth

1 onion chopped

2 cloves garlic, minced

1 teaspoon ground cumin

1/2 ground black seed

1/4 tsp cayenne pepper

3 1/2 cups cans of black beans, drain

DIRECTIONS

Heat the oil in a large pan on medium-high heat. In the pan, add onions and garlic and cook for about a minute until they are soft. After that, add the rice and simmer for about 2 minutes.

Add the vegetable broth, and make sure it is boiling. Lower the heat to a simmer and then cover the pot and cook for 20 mins.

Incorporate the black beans and sprinkle with cayenne pepper cumin and black seed powder Stir and then remove from the cooking. Allow to stand for 10 minutes prior to serving.

Sesame Spinach

This easy dish is made up of garlic, spinach along with soy sauce and black seeds. This makes it extremely healthy, and supplying you with many nutrients.

Servings: 4-6

INGREDIENTS

1 tbsp soy sauce

1 tablespoon of black seeds, toasted and crushed

1 tsp rice vinegar

1 teaspoon golden caster sugar

2 cloves of garlic grated

450g spinach, stem ends trimmed

2 tablespoons canola oil

DIRECTIONS

Add the spinach to the large pot of boiling water, and simmer for a few minutes or until the leaves begin to wilt.

Transfer the colander to a bowl then rinse it with cold water. Squeeze and drain to get rid of the most water possible. Set aside in a bowl for salad.

Then make the dressing by mixing soy sauce, oil from canola and vinegar with garlic, black seeds pepper, sugar and one small bowl. Mix well to dissolve sugar.

Serve the dressing on top of the spinach blanched and mix in a circular motion to cover

Make sure to chill for minimum one hour prior to serving.

Roasted Broccoli Salad

Servings: 4-6

INGREDIENTS

1 head broccoli, cut into florets

2 tsp lemon zest, divided

2 tablespoons lemon juice

2 cloves garlic, minced

1 teaspoon of black seeds, toast

1. 1/4 cup olive oil or more if you prefer Divided

Ground black pepper, salt and for the taste

DIRECTIONS

Heat oven until 300 degC.

in a bowl add the broccoli, one teaspoon zest of a lemon, and 1 tablespoon olive oil. Add salt and pepper according to your preference and toss well to coat.

Transfer the broccoli into an oven-proof baking dish that is lined with parchment. Then roast at 375 degrees for about 18 to 20 minutes or until golden-brown. Cool it down and then transfer into a bowl for salad.

In the meantime, toast the seeds of black in a dry pan until golden brown and fragrant. Allow them to cool.

Whisk the garlic and lemon juice within a bowl. add salt and pepper. Spread the mixture over the cooked broccoli. Sprinkle on black seeds, and stir well to mix.

Hummus With Spices

Hummus that is flavored with tomato, spices etc.

Servings: 4-6

INGREDIENTS

Freshly flavored hummus of 800g

2 tbsp olive oil

1 teaspoon black seeds

1 clove of garlic cut

1/2 tbsp. cayenne pepper

1 lime juiced

1 tomato, diced

1/2 cup of cilantro chopped

1/2 cup chopped parsley chopped

Salt and pepper are added to the taste

DIRECTIONS

Mix the hummus, garlic, tomato cayenne, black seeds herb, lime, and olive oil into the salad bowl.

Eat pita bread with it.

Main Courses

Creamy Squash Soup topped with Black Seeds

Nigella seeds provide a tasty ingredient in this soup for winter that imparts a stronger flavor, similar to the use of mustard seeds in other recipes.

Servings: 4

INGREDIENTS

2 tbsp olive oil

1 onion

2 tsp nigella seeds

A small amount of chili powder

800g squash removed, deeeded and chopped into pieces

1 potato, cubed

850 ml vegetable broth

Small bunch flat-leaf parsley

DIRECTIONS

Add olive oil into the large pot and cook on medium-high temperature. After that, add the onion. stir fry until it is golden.

Add the chili and black seeds. powder, and cook for 30 to 60 seconds.

Add the cut vegetables, squash, potato and broth, and bring the soup to a simmer.

Reduce the heat to a simmer and allow it to simmer for about 18-20 minutes, until the veggies are tender.

Blend the soup into sections, adding fresh parsley into in a blender.

Return back to the pot and let it cook for 3-4 mins.

Serve in serving bowls, and then enjoy.

Bengali Fashion Cauliflower Potato and Black Seeds

The Bengali region in India is famous for its utilization of the nigella seeds. The recipe in this recipe blends the seeds with other ingredients that are flavorful to make one of the best tasting meals you'll ever eat. (Of of course, it's difficult to flavor cauliflower--just make sure you add something flavorful to the dish. It's sort of an equivalent food item to the chalkboard.)

Servings: 34

INGREDIENTS

1 large cauliflower, cut florets

2 medium potatoes, cubed

2 tablespoons olive oil You can also make mustard oil

1 teaspoon nigella seeds

1 teaspoon mustard seeds

3-4 green chilis cut thinly

1 teaspoon sugar

1 1/2 bunch of coriander chopped

One small tomato very thinly cut

Add salt to taste

DIRECTIONS

Add the oil to a cast iron skillet and place it over medium heat. Then add the seeds of black and let them cook for 2 minutes at medium temperature until they become they are fragrant.

Add in the mustard seeds, green chili seeds and nigella seeds.

Once the seeds have slightly toasty, add the cauliflower florets in with cut potatoes. Add salt and sugar and stir it all together with a wood spoon. Cook at medium-high temperature for about 10 minutes or until the vegetables begin to turn dark around the edges.

Add 1/4 cup of water, or more if needed. lower the heat to a simmer and allow it to simmer, with the lid on, until the vegetables are soft and all liquid has evaporated. This should take about 15 minutes.

A drizzle of oil. Stir to coat. Removing from heat.

Enjoy.

Fish in Spicy Tomato Sauce

An extremely delicious and fragrant recipe bursting of Indian spices. The perfect recipe to frighten the family (especially in the case of using an entire fish head with head).

Servings: 4

INGREDIENTS

White fish fillets weighing 400-500g.

1 1/2 tsp turmeric powder

1 1/2 TSP salt to marinade

Juice from 1 lemon

1 Tbsp dried fenugreek leaf

1/2 tsp nigella seeds

1/2 teaspoon cumin seeds

8 tomatoes

2-4 chilies with greens cut finely

1 heaped tablespoon of red chilli flake

5-6 cloves of crushed garlic

1 TSP salt

A handful of cilantro chopped

DIRECTIONS

Cut the fish into chunks and put them in an empty bowl. Sprinkle with salt and turmeric powder. Drizzle with lemon juice, put the cover on and leave to rest.

3. Add 3 tablespoons of oil into a large pot and place it over a stove. Once it starts to sizzle then add the nigella, cumin seeds and fenugreek, and simmer until the seeds begin to become dark.

Chapter 15: Indian Potato And Chickpea Curry

It's as delicious as you can get. You can use it to exchange currency when you're in a financial crunch (separate in kilogram bags as well as trade in goods or services) however, some might suggest that there is no price on a dish like this.

Servings: 4

INGREDIENTS

1 can of chickpeas

2 potatoes small, chopped

1 onion diced

1 teaspoon cumin seeds

1/2 tsp nigella seeds

3 cloves

4. Black peppers

2 cm ginger, grated, or 2 tsp ginger paste

4 cloves garlic, crushed

1 tablespoon coriander powder

1 1/2 tbsp of red chilli powder

1/2 teaspoon salt, or as desired

1/4 teaspoon turmeric powder

2 tomatoes finely diced

3TBSp chopped cilantro

3-4 chilies with green chiles, cut thinly

DIRECTIONS

Add around 1/4 cup oil into the wok of a large size and set in a moderate flame. Include the black seeds, cloves, cumin seeds, peppers and cook for 1 to 2 minutes until they are fragrant.

Mix in the onion, ginger, and garlic. Fry for another 2 to 3 minutes, and then add pepper powder salt, turmeric powder and.

When the garlic and onions begin to get brown, mix in the tomatoes chopped and continue stirring until the sauce gets thicker.

Add the chopped chickpeas and potatoes. Give it an excellent stir before pouring into 1 cup of hot water. The stew should come to a simmer, and cover with a heavy lid and cooked on medium high temperatures.

Reduce the heat to a simmer and allow it to simmer until the potatoes have softened. Utilizing a spoon, break the chickpeas and potatoes for a more smoky gravy. Taste and adjust the seasonings, then take it off the stove.

Pour the soup into serving dishes and then serve with a garnish of chopped green chilies and cilantro.

Chickpea Chicken Stew

Take advantage of this tasty stew that is filled with heart-healthy nutrients and vitamins. It is great served alongside cooked basmati rice. If you're a vegetarian, or have a stance against chickens eating, you can substitute for tofu.

Servings: 4

INGREDIENT

Olive oil, coconut oil

450 g of ground chicken

1 tablespoon olive oil extra virgin

1 onion yellow, cut

2 garlic cloves diced

1 bell pepper with a green color cut into pieces

1 cup carrots, diced

1 cup celery, diced

1 (800 g) can diced tomatoes

2 (425 grams) chickpeas from a can draining

2 cups chicken broth

2 tsp black seed powder

2 teaspoons of paprika

1 teaspoon coriander

Two bay leaves

1 tablespoon red pepperflakes crushed

Add salt to taste

2TBS fresh chopped parsley

DIRECTIONS

Heat vegetable oil in a medium saucepan.

Add the chicken ground and cook for 10 minutes on medium-high temperature. Transfer the chicken to the bowl.

Then, in the pot prepare the onions and garlic until they are golden. Add carrots, celery, tomatoes as well as black seed, coriander and paprika. Add bay leaves, and red pepper flakes. Cook for about 5-8 minutes.

Transfer the chicken to the pot, then include chickpeas, chicken broth and chickpeas and cook the stew until it reaches an unbeatable simmer on low heat approximately 15 to 20 minutes.

Prior to serving, take out the bay leaves before serving and sprinkle fresh chopped parsley on top.

Enjoy.

Coconut Curry that is served with Peas and Chicken

Curry is a favorite of everyone, and this recipe using coconut milk and peas won't make any one unhappy, except for the unhappy clowns who are made to feel unhappy.

Servings: 4

INGREDIENTS

1 Tbsp brown sugar

2 Tbsp of Canola oil (divided)

3/4 cup of peas (frozen)

2 TSP curry powder (divided)

3 medium potatoes (cut)

1 cup of carrots (sliced)

One large onion (chopped)

3/4 teaspoon salt (divided)

1 tsp nigella seeds (black seed)

1 (400 grams) 1 (400 g) "light" coconut milk

1 (400 grams) is a reduced-sodium chicken broth

1 tablespoon garlic (chopped)

700g of boneless and skinless, and skinless chicken breast (cut in cubes)

1 cup of celery (chopped)

1/4 cup fresh cilantro (chopped)

DIRECTIONS

Place the cut chicken pieces in the bowl and sprinkle with 1 1/4 salt, and 1 teaspoon the black seed paste. Mix it all together with your hands until coated.

Add 1 teaspoon of oil into the large pot and cook on medium-high heat. Put the chicken that has been seasoned inside the pan. Roast at least a couple of times until the chicken is an all-over golden crust around 8 to 9 minutes. Take the chicken out of the pan and put aside.

Add the rest of 1 tablespoon of oil into the pot, fry onions and garlic and nigella seeds until toasty approximately 3 minutes.

Add 1 teaspoon curry powder. Cook for one minute or so, until the curry powder is fragrant.

Add the celery, potatoes, coconut milk and carrots broth, and remaining 1/2 teaspoon salt. boil over high heat with frequent stirring. When it starts to boil then reduce the temperature to low and allow it to simmer, with a stirring interval until the potatoes and carrots are softened for 8 to 10 minutes.

Put the chicken back into the pan, and stir into the peas. Increase the heat to high and cook another 5 minutes or until the chicken has cooked to your liking.

Sweet Potato, Carrot, and Red Lentil Soup

The hot red lentil soup is perfect for any time. The combination of cilantro and carrots gives a lovely colour and a fresh appearance to the soup. Be careful not to spill it on your white shirts, in case someone might think you cut yourself.

Servings: 6-8

INGREDIENTS

Two tablespoons of olive oil

1 big sweet yellow onion chopped into pieces

One large sweet potato cut into chunks and peeled.

5-6 large carrots that have been chopped and peeled (about four cups)

1 cup of red lentils

8 cups vegetable stock

1 tablespoon Harissa paste

2 teaspoons Ras el Hanout

1 teaspoon of salt

1 teaspoon of pepper

Nigella seeds for garnish

Cilantro cut into pieces, to use as garnish

DIRECTIONS

Warm the olive oil on the large griddle on moderate heat. Incorporate the onions and cook in a couple of minutes until soft and translucent, approximately 7 minutes.

Add the carrots lentils, potatoes harissa paste, sal and pepper. Pour in the stock of vegetables and heat to.

Reduce the temperature and simmer under cover with a lid, until the lentils, carrots, and potatoes are soft about 20-25 minutes. Removing the pan from the stove and let it cool.

Blend soup in small sections until it is smooth and creamy. Taste and adjust seasonings.

Pour the soup in serving bowls. Add chopped cilantro, black seeds, and chopped cilantro and then enjoy.

Persian Mushroom Stew

If you've failed geography. Persian signifies regionally Iranian.

Servings: 4-6

INGREDIENTS

900g of mushrooms, cut into slices

3 tablespoons of vegetable oil

1 onion, cut

2 garlic cloves diced

1 teaspoon of black seeds powdered with

1 teaspoon black cumin powder

Salt, peppers according to your preference

2 tablespoons of flour

1. 1 Cup almond milk

DIRECTIONS

Heat the oil on a pan. In the skillet, add the onion and garlic and sauté for 2 minutes before adding the mushrooms.

Reduce the heat down to low, and cook the mushrooms with their juices for about 10 minutes.

Mix the flour with milk, then pour it into the pan and over the mushrooms.

Let it cook until it starts to thicken, then alter the flavor with spices like salt, pepper or the cumin powder.

Remove the pot from the heat, and serve warm.

Roasted vegetables with Lamb

Servings: 4

INGREDIENTS

1 tbsp olive oil

250g of lean lamb fillet Thinly cut

140g shallots, halved

2 large zucchinis cut into chunks

1/2 tsp black seed powder

1/2 teaspoon ground coriander

Three bell peppers (of various shades) Cut

1 clove of garlic, cut into slices

3/4 cup vegetable stock

1 cup cherry tomatoes

A handful of cilantro leaves cut

Salt, pepper and salt

DIRECTIONS

Add the oil in an enormous saucepan, then set at a high temperature.

Add the shallots, garlic and lamb to the pan and simmer for 3-4 minutes, until they are golden.

In the meantime, add the zucchinis. cook for approximately 5 minutes or until they are cooked. Mix in the black seed powder as well as coriander.

Add the peppers and garlic, decrease the heat to medium, and cook for approximately 5 minutes, until the peppers become soft.

Add the tomatoes along with vegetable broth, and let it simmer in a covered pot for between 12 and 15 minutes, mixing often.

Serve the dish sprinkled with coarsely chopped cilantro before serving.

Traditional Winter Stew featuring Chickpeas and Vegetables

It is a delicious combination of vegetables and spices. Also, it's rich in vitamins and proteins. It is very satisfying and ideal to eat for dinner or lunch. There are no adverse effects when you consume it during the winter months rather than during summer.

Servings: 8

INGREDIENTS

2 teaspoons olive oil

1. 1 Cup chopped onions

1 cup (1/2-inch) slices leek

1/2 teaspoon ground coriander

1/2 teaspoon crushed black seeds

1/8 tsp black cumin ground

1/8 teaspoon red pepper, crushed

1 clove of garlic, crushed

3 1/3 cups vegetable stock divided into 3 portions

Two cups (1-inch) butternut squash cut, peeled

1 Cup (1/2-inch) carrots sliced

3/4 cup (1-inch) Yukon gold potato, peeled, cubed

1 tablespoon harissa

1 1/2 tsp tomato paste

3/4 teaspoon salt

450 g of turnips peeled and cut into 8 wedges

1 (430 grams) can chickpeas, rinsed

1/4 cup fresh flat-leaf parsley, chopped

1 1/2 tsp honey

1 1/3 cups uncooked couscous

Chapter 16: Eight Lemon Wedges

DIRECTIONS

Add the olive oil into the pot in a large bowl and place on medium-high heat.

Add leeks as well as onions and cook for five minutes. Add the black seeds and cumin, coriander, red pepper, garlic and stir-fry for about one moment.

Incorporate the butternut squash potatoes, carrots, tomato paste harissa, turnips, and salt. Add 3 cups vegetable stock and bring to a simmer.

Reduce the heat, then let it simmer with a lid for approximately 30 minutes.

Mix sugar and parsley chopped.

2. Take 2/3 cup of cooking liquid hot of the butternut squash soup and pour it into the bowl of a medium size. Add the 2/3 cup of stock in addition.

Mix in the couscous. mix and allow to sit for five minutes in a covered. Fluff the couscous using an fork.

The stew can be served on top of the couscous that has been cooked, and sprinkle with freshly cut cilantro leaves.

Serve it with wedges of lemon.

Fried Chicken Stuffed With Rice

The delicious chicken can be enjoyed with almonds, rice raisins and cherries. If you're vegan, replace your chicken for pepper or eggplant. However, it would make for a completely different dish to that point. (Still good, though).

Servings8

INGREDIENTS

One whole chicken

2 TSP salt

2 large onions carefully sliced

3 cloves of garlic

1. 1 Tablespoon olive oil

1/2 cup long-grain rice

1/4 teaspoon of black seed powder

1/4 teaspoon cardamom

1/4 tsp of cinnamon

1 cup chicken stock

1 cup of sour cherries that have been soaked and then drained

4 Tbsp of sliced almonds

3 tbsp raisins

2 Tbsp freshly squeezed lime juice

1/4 cup juice from apples

DIRECTIONS

Rinse the chicken thoroughly and rub dry. Place 1 tablespoon of oil in a large skillet on moderate flame. Add the garlic and onions and sauté for 3-5 mins until the onions are golden caramelized.

Add the cooked rice, the cinnamon and black seeds, cardamom 1, 1 teaspoon salt, and pepper. Cook for 5 more minutes, mixing frequently.

Then, add the chicken broth, and slow cook for about 12-15 minutes. Cover.

Add the sour cherry, raisins the almonds as well as lime juice, and then remove the skillet from the heat. Adjust the seasoning according to your preference.

Place the rice mixture inside the cavity of the chicken, and then securely tie the legs of the chicken.

Sprinkle with 1 teaspoon of salt, one pinch cinnamon and black seed powder. 1 teaspoon sugar, and apply a coating to evenly.

Put the chicken stuffed on a baking tray, sprinkle the apple juice on top of the chicken, then cover it with foil, then roast within the oven, for about 45 minutes.

Enjoy!

Tasty mystery Stew With Green Beans and potatoes

The ingredient that is mysterious that is a mystery ingredient (spoiler)--nigella seeds.

Servings: 10

INGREDIENTS

450 g green beans, cut

1 tbsp olive oil

1 onion, cut

1/2 tbsp nigella seeds

1 (800 grams) could be whole plum tomatoes and juice or fresh tomatoes

2 zucchinis, cut into half moons

Garlic, Cayenne oregano, and thyme for enjoy the taste

One large potato cleaned and chopped into cubes

Black and salt To be tasted

Freshly chopped parsley

DIRECTIONS

Add olive oil into an enormous saucepan, and place at a moderate flame. In the meantime, add the onion and the seeds of nigella and cook for about 3-4 minutes until the onion becomes soft and golden.

Include the green beans, stir and cook for five minutes. Add the zucchini pieces tomato, potatoes, potatoes and garlic. Season by adding the cayenne oregano and thyme. salt, and pepper.

When the stew is beginning to simmer, lower the temperature and cook, with the lid on, for around 20 minutes, or until the potatoes begin to soften.

Pour the stew into an serving bowl. Sprinkle with freshly chopped parsley, and serve with bread that has been toasted.

Servings: 4-6

INGREDIENTS

2 Tbsp vegetable oil

900 grams fresh mushrooms, chopped

2 cups can of black beans, drain

1 onion cut into slices

4 cloves of garlic, diced

1 cup tomato puree

5 cups vegetable stock

1 TSP black seed powder

2 potatoes cut and peeled

1/4 tsp cayenne pepper

1. 1/4 cup diced cilantro

Salt and pepper to your taste

DIRECTIONS

Add the vegetable oil to an oven-proof saucepan. Set it over the medium flame.

Incorporate the onion and garlic. Cook for 2 minutes and after which add the mushrooms cayenne pepper, and potatoes. Cook for 5 more minutes.

Rinse the beans, then put them in the pot alongside the puree of tomatoes. Add the vegetable stock and heat to a simmer over an extremely high heat.

Then reduce the heat to medium and simmer it for 20 to 25 minutes or until the vegetables are soft and the stew is somewhat increased in thickness.

Stir in chopped cilantro. serve.

Barley Soup with vegetable

Barley is a great source of nutrition with a very high amount and has a rich, nutty taste which is great for soups as well as salads and stews.

Servings: 4-6

INGREDIENTS:

2 tablespoons olive oil

1 onion, cut

1 clove of garlic, cut

1 cup of uncooked barley washed

4 cups vegetable stock

1/2 tsp black seed powder

1 1/2 tsp normal (black cumin) powder

1 lime juiced

2 tomatoes, diced

1 carrot, diced

Salt and pepper to the taste

1 tablespoon chopped parsley

450g of chicken chopped

DIRECTIONS

Warm the olive oil inside a pot that is set on medium flame. Place the chicken in the pan and cook each side for 10 minutes. Then remove the chicken from the pan.

Add oil to the pot and cook the onions and garlic for 2 minutes, then mix in the barley as well as black seed powder, and cumin.

Cook for another 2 minutes, then mix in the carrot and tomatoes.

Add the stock and sprinkle with salt and pepper, and Bring to a boil. Lower the heat to a simmer before transferring the chicken to the pot and allow it to simmer for 20 minutes, or until the vegetables are soft and the meat is cooked to perfection..

Mix into the chopped parsley. pour into serving bowl, and then enjoy.

Serve it warm and fresh.

Shepherd's Pie with Cumin and black Seeds

It's a delicious and spicy shepherd's pies made of ground meat and cauliflower. The whole family will enjoy it If you're not scared of strange ingredients such as black cumin, which you find on strange cookbooks that you discover into the midnight on Amazon.com.

Servings: 6

INGREDIENTS

2 Tbsp butter, 1/2 1 tsp of pepper

1/2 teaspoon black cumin powder

1/2 teaspoon of black seed powder

1 onion that has been minced finely

2 Tbsp lemon juice

1kg ground beef

1 1/2 tbsp olive oil

1 3/4 cups cheddar cheese (grated)

1 TSP salt

2 small cauliflowers

DIRECTIONS

Preheat oven to 170 degrees Celsius and then lightly coat the baking pan with oil.

Boil the cauliflower in the pot of boiling water until it becomes soft approximately 15 minutes.

In a deep frying pan, heat olive oil. Cook the steak until brown. After that, sprinkle with salt black seed powder, and pepper and cook it at least 20-22 minutes.

Add the onion and cook for the remaining three to four minutes. Pour the mixture of beef and onions with lemon juice. Give it an additional stir before transferring onto the pan that you prepared. The beef mixture should be spread evenly.

In a bowl mix the cauliflower in butter. Spread it on top of the beef. Sprinkle the cauliflower with cheese, then cook in the oven about 15 to 20 minutes. Set aside for a minimum of 5 minutes before serving.

Chapter 17: Vegetable-Beef Stir Fry

The following recipe will require you to be sure to follow the steps of the preparation process in the direction. If not, the result can be disastrous. Like most people, if you're vegan or vegetarian substitute tofu for beef.

Servings: 2-4

INGREDIENTS

2 tbsp olive oil

1/2 tsp red bell pepper Flakes

1/4 cup of green onion, cut thinly

1/4 cup soy sauce

215 grams boneless beef sirloin

2 cloves of garlic, chopped

1 cup broccoli, cut into slices

1/2 tsp black seed powder

1/2 teaspoon ground cumin

2 Tbsp cooking oil

1 tablespoon sugar

1 cup of chopped cauliflower florets

1/3 cup chilled water

1 tablespoon cornstarch

1/2 teaspoon pepper

1 cup carrot, peeled, julienned

DIRECTIONS

Slice the beef thinly and then place it in a bowl that is large. Include the soy sauce, onions and red pepper flakes garlic, olive oil, sugar. Season with the ground black pepper. Gently mix until well-mixed.

Allow the beef to marinate for 30 to 40 minutes at temperatures of room temperature.

After that, drain the meat, and save the marinade to be used later.

In a small glass mix the cornstarch with water. Stir into the marinade, and add the black seed powder.

1. Add one tablespoon cooking oil to a large fry pan, and place it over the flame to cook. Then add the carrots, and cook for 3-4 mins, making sure to stir often.

Add the cauliflower as well as broccoli, and cook for two to three minutes, or until the veggies become tender.

Transfer the vegetables into an additional dish and cover with a lid to keep warm.

Add the rest of the oil in the pan, and place on medium-high temperature. After that, stir fry the meat in two batches until golden brown all over.

Add all of the beef ingredients in the pan. Add the cornstarch and heat to a boil until the sauce has thickened and stirs regularly.

Incorporate the vegetables and simmer for another 5 minutes, then take the dish off of the stove.

Serve with rice that is hot.

Healthy and Flavorful Pumpkin Soup

It's a delicious healthy and nutritious soup. It is chock loaded with spices. It can be made in a matter of minutes. Kids will be delighted. Be careful not to let them read the word "healthy" in the recipe name.

Servings: 4

INGREDIENTS

2 teaspoons extra olive oil

900g of pumpkin removed and seeds

2 leeks, cut and then sliced

1 clove garlic crushed

1 TSP black or regular cumin ground

1 teaspoon of black seeds, toast

3. 3 Cups vegetable stock (or water

Salt, according to your be tasted

Black pepper to be tasted

DIRECTIONS

Use a sharp knife to remove the pumpkin, then cut into pieces that are coarse. In the large pot and cook on a medium-high temperature.

Add the leeks, as well as garlic to the pan, then cook until soft.

Add the cumin. Cook for a further minutes. Then add the pumpkin pieces add the stock or water then sprinkle on salt and pepper and cook on a low temperature.

If it starts to be boiling, lower the temperature to a simmering level of about 25 to 30 minutes or until the pumpkin is soft. Transfer the soup into an blender, and blend until it is pureed.

Return the soup in the pan and simmer for about a minute. Distribute the soup into serving bowls. Sprinkle with black seeds, and serve right away.

Baked Rice with Spinach, Coconut Milk

I'm sure I'm supposed to add more vegan-friendly recipes to this post. Here's another I think is a good start.

Servings: 10

INGREDIENTS

Three tablespoons a nutritious oil of your choice

1 teaspoon of pepper

1 cup long rice

2 (13 1/2 oz.) coconut milk cans

2 teaspoons black seed powder

1 cup of onion chopped

1 1/2 teaspoon salt

2 (280 grams) packs of spinach frozen (thawed then chopped)

2 cups brown lentils cooked

2 cloves of garlic minced

DIRECTIONS

Heat oven until 175°C.

The oil should be added in an oven-proof dish and place it over a low flame. In the pan, add onion and garlic and cook until golden.

Add black seeds, powder and rice. Season with pepper and salt, and cook for a further 3 minutes.

Mix in the cooked lentils and spinach as well as pouring into the coconut milk mix. Cover with a lid and place in the oven.

Bake 35-40 mins, until the top is light gold. Serve right away.

Baked Goods

Nigella Flatbread

It is important to note that these recipes do not have anything to be associated in any way with Nigella Lawson. It's not like I'm calling her"flatbread," although I could "flatbread", although it could be tempting to use that term.

Six breads are made.

INGREDIENTS

to bake bread

2 tablespoons olive oil (plus additional greasing)

15g/1 tablespoon freshly baked yeast

1 Tbsp plain yoghurt

500 grams of white, strong bread flour

2 teaspoons of salt

2 tablespoons plain yoghurt

300ml of warm water

to refer to the glaze

1 large egg

1 teaspoon of water

1 tbsp nigella seeds

DIRECTIONS

Combine the yeast, flour and salt into the large mixing bowl. Create a hole in the middle. In a small dish, combine the yogurt with oil. Mix in the water, then blend thoroughly.

Mix the ingredients into the flour mix and stir with a spoon until you have a soft dough.

The dough should be transferred to the work surface that has been dusted and gently knead the dough with your hands. If you find the dough to be sticky, add more flour until the dough becomes flexible.

Form your dough into a huge ball, then coat it with oil, then place it in an empty bowl. Place it in an unclean kitchen towel, and allow it to rest for an hour or so to rise.

After the dough is increased in size, cut the dough into six pieces.

After that, using the rolling pin, form each ball into an oval-shaped thin strip. Set them out on two baking sheets. Let them remain for fifteen minutes wrapped in kitchen towels.

With your hands or kitchen knives create diagonal lines on the breads, then trace identical lines on the other side in order to create a criss-cross design.

In a smaller dish, mix the egg using yogurt and water. Brush the mix on sandwich bread.

Dust with nigella seeds, then bake in the oven preheated to 180 C until the crust is golden brown and soft to the touch.

Remove the cake from the oven, and then take a bite to.

Nigella Walnut Shortbread

Is it unhappy that it's known as "short"?

Makes 25

INGREDIENTS

250g of butter softened

1/2 teaspoon vanilla extract

1 1/4 cup plain flour

1. 1/4 cup corn meal

1 teaspoon of ground black seeds

1 teaspoon lemon juice

3/4 salt

1/4 cup walnuts minced finely

1 egg lightly beat

Chapter 18: Sea Salt Flakes

Freshly ground black

DIRECTIONS

Pre-heat oven to 180C. Two baking sheets should be lined with baking papers.

Combine all the ingredients, including cornflour vanilla, flour, black seeds, lemon juice as well as salt into the bowl of a large one and mix using an electric mixer to make dough.

Make sure to dust your work area with flour, then place the dough on top. Work the dough with your hands, then make two balls.

Use the rolling pin to roll your dough to form a fine circle. Cut the dough using the cookie cutter that is round. Spread the cookies on the baking sheets.

Repeat this process for the second dough ball. Put the cookies in the refrigerator and let them rest for around half an time.

Whisk eggs in a small bowl, then apply the egg wash over top of the cookies.

Then, sprinkle them with sea salt as well as black pepper. Bake them in the oven for about 18 to 20 minutes, until they are the cookies are golden.

Take them out of the oven. Cool them for about 15 minutes before enjoying.

Nigella Seed Cookies

It makes about 36 cookies

INGREDIENTS

1.5 cup whole wheat flour

1 cup all-purpose flour

1/4 cup semolina

1tsp. baking powder

1tsp. salt

1tsp. sugar

2 tsp. nigella seeds

1 stick of butter softened

1/4 cup milk

DIRECTIONS

Preheat oven at 175 degC.

Mix the entire wheat flour all-purpose flour semolina and baking powder and salt, as well as sugar in one large bowl. Mix very well.

Add the softened butter to blend with your hands until it is like fine crumbles.

Mix the milk in slowly at a time until you get a soft dough. Place on a surface that is floured and, using a rolling pin form a fine circular.

Cut them into round or different shapes using the cookie cutter. Place the pieces on baking dishes that is lined with parchment.

Repeat until the dough is gone. Bake the dough in the oven for approximately 25 minutes or until the dough is rising and slightly firm.

Mini Mushroom, Kalonji and Feta Pies

Servings 6

INGREDIENTS

To fill the jar:

500g Portobello mushrooms, sliced

100g feta cheese, crumbled

1 Tbsp butter

3 cloves garlic, crushed

1/2 teaspoon black seeds

1 tsp lemonyme

1/2 teaspoon black pepper

Crust

Plain flour 235g

55ml of water

50ml skimmed milk

Unsalted Butter 75g

1 TSP salt

Mixture of milk and turmeric to apply a paste on the pastry caps

DIRECTIONS

Heat the butter in an oven over moderate heat. In the skillet, add the garlic and black seeds. Fry for 1-2 minutes, until the garlic is golden and fragrant. Cook the mushrooms for five minutes. mix in the thyme. add black pepper, and take the heat off.

Transfer to a colander to drain. When cool enough for handling then squeeze the mushroom mixture by using hands to get rid of the most liquid possible. Mix in the feta, and let it sit for at least 20 minutes.

Pre-heat the oven to 160°C.

To prepare the dough, mix butter, milk and the water in a large saucepan, and heat to the point of boiling.

Mix in the flour. Mix thoroughly and then transfer onto a surface that has been dusted with flour. Use your hands to knead until the dough is completely smooth.

Make 6 balls. Then reserve 1/3 of each to be used to make a lid for pies. The balls should be rolled into a circular shape and then put them in an ice cream tin. pressing with fingers until both the sides and bottom are fully covered.

Pour about 2 tablespoons of mushrooms into each muffin cup. Make the dough balls, then top the pie by pressing them against the edges using fingers to secure.

Warm the milk inside a saucepan Add turmeric and stir well before brushing the mixture on the pies.

Bake the cake in the oven preheated for 35 to 40 minutes. Enjoy.

Indian Potato Stuffed Bread (Kulcha)

It's a quick and delicious dish for Kulcha or Indian bread that is stuffed with stuffing. What could be better to make with bread than stuffing things inside it? (I've been wanting to remain "stuff stuff").

Servings: 8

INGREDIENTS

For stuffing

2 pieces large cooked potatoes

1 onion chopped

2-3 pieces of green chilies, cut

1/4 teaspoon turmeric powder

1/4 teaspoon salt

Bread for breakfast

1 cup all-purpose flour

Oil refined used to cook with

1/4 tablespoon nigella seeds

1 tablespoon of coriander leaves

3 tablespoons curd

Chapter 19: Two Cups Of Buttermilk

1 large egg

3 Tbsp vegetable oil

1-1/2 cups yellow self-rising cornmeal

2 cups sharp shredded Cheddar cheese

1 tsp nigella seeds

DIRECTIONS

Preheat oven to 230 degrees C. Make sure you grease the rim of a square or round baking dish using vegetable oil, and put it in the oven for five minutes, until it is heated properly.

Toast a handful of seeds of nigella, using the traditional toasting of nigella seeds method.

In a medium bowl, mix the cornmeal, egg, buttermilk, and cheese. Next, mix in the seeds. Mix well, and then pour the mix into the pan.

Bake the corn bread for at 25 minutes. Allow it to stand in the pan 5 minutes before cutting into slices and serve.

Black Seed Flavored Flatbreads

Flavorful and delicious flatbreads made from fresh ingredients. They are flavoured by toasted black seeds. It is a breeze to prepare.

Servings: 8

INGREDIENTS

1 1/4 cup natural yogurt

12 a pinch of salt

400g of all-purpose flour. Add another to dust

1 tablespoon the black seeds, toast

DIRECTIONS

The grill should be heated to medium. Prepare a baking dish by coating it with flour. In a large bowl, mix the seeds of black and flour add the salt and a pinch. Add the yogurt, as well as 1/3 cup of wate.

Mix well until you have a soft dough.

Divide into 8 parts. Each ball into circles or ovals and then place them on the baking sheet.

Sprinkle lightly with flour. Grill at least 4-5 minutes each portion until lightly brown and well-puffed. Serve hot.

Black Seed Cupcakes

It only takes about an hour to create these delicious cupcakes. Have them while sipping the coffee or tea.

Servings: 12

INGREDIENTS

1 cup all-purpose flour

1. 1 tablespoon baking powder

1 teaspoon salt

1. 1/4 cup baking soda

2 tablespoons butter

1 Tbsp olive oil extra-light oil

1 cup of Granulated sugar

1 large egg

1 large white egg

2 Tbsp lemonrind, grated

1 cup buttermilk

2 Tbsp of black seeds

DIRECTIONS

Heat oven until 175 degrees Celsius. Sprinkle 12 muffin cups in cooking spray or line them with parchment paper.

Mix the oil and butter in a bowl, and mix thoroughly, adding gradually the sugar granulated. Make sure to beat it thoroughly. Include one egg. Followed by the white of the egg.

Then, add the lemon's the rind. In a separate bowl mix the baking powder, flour along with salt, soda in the egg mix.

Mix with the seeds of black.

Pour the mix into muffin cups. Bake within the oven 20 to 22 minutes, or until A toothpick placed into the middle is free of any traces. Place the pan on an air-tight rack and let it let it cool.

Enjoy.

Cheddar Scones

The book is finished by eating Scones. Cheddar cheese as well as black seeds combine in this healthy recipe to provide an amazing taste. We'll be back soon!

Servings: 12-14

INGREDIENTS

400 g of all-purpose flour

4 tbsp natural low fat yogurt

4 tsp of xanthan gum

150 g of butter

2 tsp baking soda

2 tsp dijon mustard

Salt Pinch

80 g potato starch

2 large eggs, beate

2 TSP black seeds

3 1/2 oz. (100 grams) cheddar grated

1/2 cup (100ml) milk

DIRECTIONS

Heat the oven to 220 degree Celsius. Prepare a baking sheet with paper.

In a bowl, mix the flour, cornstarch baking soda, butter, and xanthan gum. Add salt to taste and stir it well. Stir with the cheese grated and the black seeds.